# DR. NC ... 1200-CALORIE DIET PLAN

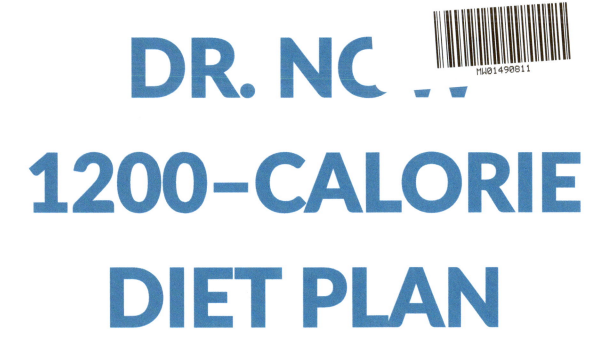

## *EMPOWER YOUR*

## *WEIGHT LOSS JOURNEY*

### 1200-CALORIE DIET WITH LOW-COST RECIPES

### STEP-BY-STEP GUIDANCE

### 7-DAY KICK-START DETOX MEAL PLAN
### +
### 30-DAY SUPPORTIVE MEAL PLAN

***

Magda Tangy

## CHAPTER 7: MAIN DISHES

# INTRODUCTION

Welcome to "The Dr. Now 1200-Calorie Diet Plan: Empower Your Weight Loss Journey"!
In this book, we will embark on a transformative journey towards achieving significant weight loss and improving your overall health. Through a combination of low-cost recipes, step-by-step guidance, and a supportive plan, you will gain the tools and knowledge needed to succeed.

As a seasoned health and wellness writer, I understand the difficulties and frustrations that frequently accompany weight loss attempts.
That's why I've crafted this book to be your personal guide, providing clear and actionable steps to simplify the complex world of nutrition and weight loss.
By following this 1200-calorie diet plan, you can achieve sustainable long-term results and reduce health risks associated with obesity.

However, this book isn't solely focused on the numbers on the scale. It's designed to empower you to whip up positive changes in your life. I will be your supportive coach, addressing your concerns, managing your expectations, and encouraging you to believe in your capacity for change.

So let's begin this journey together. Get ready to discover practical meal plans, overcome common frustrations, and find the motivation you need to achieve your weight loss goals.
Remember, you are capable of transforming your life, and I'm here to guide you every step of the way.

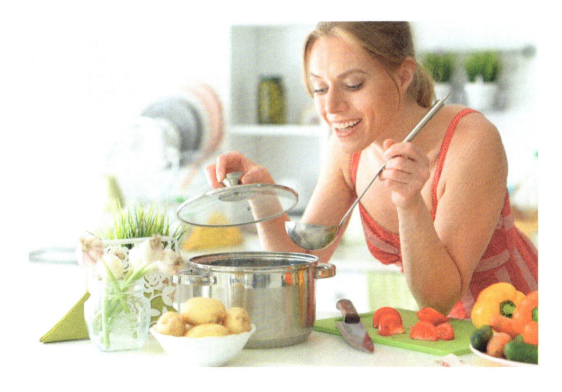

# CHAPTER 1: WELCOME TO YOUR WEIGHT LOSS JOURNEY

Starting to lose weight isn't just about losing a few pounds; it's also about making big changes to how you live your life. This chapter will help you get ready for success by looking at what drives you, setting attainable goals, encouraging a positive attitude, and creating long-lasting habits in a helpful setting.

## 1.1 CLARIFYING YOUR "WHY"

Think about the reasons you want to lose weight. Getting clear on your "why" is important whether you want to improve your health, get more energy, or feel more confident. It will boost your motivation and help you stay on track.

> **Actionable Step:** Record your weight loss goals and place them in a location where you will frequently see them—such as on your phone's lock screen, your refrigerator, or your bathroom mirror.

## 1.2 SETTING REALISTIC EXPECTATIONS

Losing weight calls for time and commitment. Sometimes, being let down by high hopes when things don't go as fast as you had hoped can happen. Establishing achievable objectives, on the other hand, allows you to savor minor victories and maintain your progress.

**Focus on Sustainable Changes:** Aim for steady, incremental progress instead of pursuing immediate results. Long-term success requires you to create habits that will last.

**Celebrate Small Victories:** Every tiny step forward holds significance. Remember that not all changes show up on the scale. Positive outcomes include increased vitality, improved sleep quality, and a generalized sense of strength.

> **Actionable Steps:** Divide your major objective into doable steps for you. For example, set a goal to lose 5 pounds in the first month or work out every day for 10 minutes. At each milestone, reward yourself with something special that isn't food. For example, read a new book, take a relaxing bath, or plan a fun trip.

## 1.3 CULTIVATING A POSITIVE MINDSET

Having a good attitude is essential if you want to lose weight. It's not just what you eat or how much you work out; it's also how you think and how you deal with problems as they come up.

**Focus on Progress, Not Perfection:** Stress how important it is to keep making progress instead of trying to be perfect. Remember that challenges are a natural part of the process and can provide valuable lessons. Embrace obstacles as opportunities for growth and understanding. Note every victory you have—no matter how little—then let them inspire you to press on.

**Practice Self-Compassion:** Know that reducing weight is difficult and that occasionally things won't go as expected. Show the same friendliness you would want in place of self-criticism. Thank you for your efforts; enjoy your successes and pardon yourself for any mistakes.

**Stay Present with Mindfulness:** Try to make things like meditation, deep breathing, and eating with awareness a part of your daily life. These habits can help you recognize when you're hungry or full, figure out what makes you eat when you're upset, and make decisions that help you reach your goals.

> **Actionable Step:** Start with a daily mindfulness exercise, like spending five minutes focusing on your breathing or doing a body scan to notice any areas of tension. Use these moments to reset your mindset and reinforce positive self-talk.

## 1.4 BUILDING HEALTHY HABITS AND CREATING A SUPPORTIVE ENVIRONMENT

Effective weight loss is about creating long-term sustainable habits rather than about deprivation. Your surroundings have a big impact on these habits.

**Adopt Small, Manageable Changes:** Begin by identifying small changes you can incorporate into your daily routine, such as eating balanced meals, getting regular exercise, and staying hydrated. Little changes taken together will have significant long-term advantages.

**Create a Supportive Environment:** Do your best to be around positive, encouraging individuals who will cheer you on while you pursue your ambitions. This could include family members, friends, or online communities who share a similar journey. Additionally, create a home environment that fosters success by stocking your pantry with healthy foods, preparing meals in advance, and minimizing temptations.

> **Actionable Steps:** Define specific, quantifiable, attainable, relevant, and time-bound goals.
>
> For example, rather than saying, "I want to lose weight," define your goal more specifically: "I will lose 10 pounds in three months by following a 1200-calorie diet and walking for 30 minutes five times a week."
>
> Create a daily routine that includes time for meal planning, exercise, self-care, and relaxation. Consistency is key to building new habits.
>
> Join a support group, partner with a weight loss buddy, or seek out online communities for motivation and accountability.

**Conclusion: Start with a Strong Mindset**

By understanding your "why," setting realistic expectations, cultivating a positive mindset, and building healthy habits in a supportive environment, you are laying a solid foundation for success. This isn't just about reducing weight; it's about being the best version of yourself—healthier and happier. You need to be patient, optimistic, and focused on making progress.

# CHAPTER 2: THE SCIENCE BEHIND THE DR. NOW DIET

Grasping the principles of the Dr. Now 1200-Calorie Diet Plan is crucial to appreciating its effectiveness in promoting weight loss and enhancing overall health. This chapter will break down the core principles of the diet—caloric deficit, balanced nutrition, and strategic macronutrient distribution—to give you a clear understanding of how and why this plan works.

## 2.1 HOW THE 1200-CALORIE DIET WORKS

The Dr. Now 1200-Calorie Diet is based on several core principles that work together to promote weight loss and improve overall health. By following this structured plan, you can achieve a sustainable caloric deficit, maintain balanced nutrition, and ensure long-term success.

**Caloric Deficit:** The basis of the Dr. Now Diet entails creating a caloric deficit, which occurs when you consume fewer calories than your body needs to maintain its present weight. By following a strict daily calorie intake of 1200 calories, you set up your body to burn fat stores for energy, which leads to weight loss.

.

**Macronutrient Balance:** The diet focuses on a deliberate balance of macronutrients (proteins, carbs, and fats) to promote weight loss while maintaining general health.

- **High Protein:** Helps preserve muscle mass, which is important for a healthy metabolism, and promotes satiety (feeling full), reducing overall calorie intake. The emphasis is on lean protein sources such as fish, poultry, tofu, lentils, and low-fat dairy products.
- **Low Carbohydrates:** Limits refined carbohydrates and sugars to control blood sugar levels and promote fat burning. Focuses on complex carbohydrates, like whole grains, vegetables, and fruits, to provide sustained energy and reduce cravings.
- **Low Fat:** Encourages moderation in fat intake, specifically reducing saturated and trans fats that can contribute to heart disease. Recommends eating healthy fats that don't interfere with weight loss efforts, such as those found in avocados, nuts, seeds, and olive oil.

**Hydration:** Staying hydrated is essential for the success of this diet plan. Drinking at least 8 cups (64 ounces) of water daily supports digestion, metabolic processes, and helps control hunger. Incorporating herbal teas or flavored water can also help maintain hydration levels.

## 2.2 COMMON MYTHS AND FACTS ABOUT LOW-CALORIE DIETS

Low-calorie diets, like the Dr. Now 1200-Calorie Diet, often come with misconceptions that can deter people from following them. Let's clarify some common myths and provide facts to support you in making wise decisions:

**Myth: Low-calorie diets are ineffective for weight loss.**
**Fact:** Low-calorie diets, when properly managed, can be incredibly effective by creating a calorie deficit. This process compels the body to burn stored fat for energy.

**Myth: Low-calorie diets slow down your metabolism.**
**Fact:** While metabolism may slow down temporarily with reduced calorie intake, this effect is usually not significant enough to prevent weight loss. The diet's emphasis on high protein and muscle maintenance helps mitigate this effect.

**Myth: Low-calorie diets cause muscle loss.**
**Fact:** Including adequate protein in your meals, such as chicken, fish, tofu, and legumes, helps minimize muscle loss while promoting fat loss.

**Myth: Low-calorie diets lead to nutrient deficiencies.**
**Fact:** When properly planned, low-calorie diets can provide all necessary nutrients. The Dr. Now Diet Plan emphasizes meals high in nutrients to meet your body's nutritional needs.

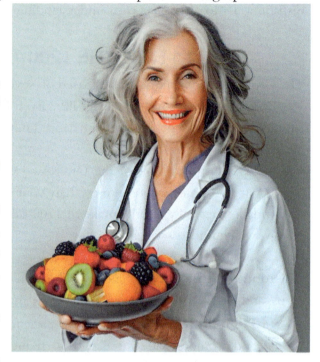

**Myth: Low-calorie diets are too restrictive and unsustainable.**
**Fact:** The Dr. Now 1200-Calorie Diet Plan is designed to be practical and sustainable, with a variety of low-cost recipes and step-by-step guidance to make weight loss achievable and enjoyable.

**Conclusion: Understanding the Science for Success**
By understanding the principles of the Dr. Now 1200-Calorie Diet—caloric deficit, balanced nutrition, and mindful macronutrient distribution—you are better equipped to follow the plan and achieve your weight loss goals. This diet is not just about reducing calorie intake; it's about making healthier food choices and fostering sustainable habits for long-term health improvements.

# CHAPTER 3: PRACTICAL TIPS FOR DIET SUCCESS

Embarking on a weight loss journey is simpler with the right mindset, tools, and strategies. This chapter includes practical recommendations to help you remain on track with the Dr. Now 1200-Calorie Diet Plan, including effective meal prepping, smart shopping, and mastering portion control.

## 3.1 PREPARING FOR SUCCESS: STOCKING AND PREPPING

Success on the Dr. Now 1200-Calorie Diet Plan starts with having a well-prepared kitchen and pantry. The right ingredients and tools will make it easier to prepare healthy meals and avoid temptation. By combining smart stocking and meal planning practices, you may save time, minimize stress, and guarantee that you always have healthful options available.

**Clear Out Unhealthy Foods:** Begin by removing or donating any high-calorie, processed foods, sugary snacks, and drinks that do not align with your weight loss goals. Clearing out these items reduces temptation and creates space for healthier alternatives.

**Create a Food-Free Space:** Establish a Food-Free Zone: Decide which parts of your house, like the living room or bedroom, are off limits to eating.
This can help break the habit of mindless snacking and create a healthier relationship with food.

**Stock Up on Nutrient-Dense Staples:** Fill your pantry with foods that support your diet plan:
- **Whole Grains:** Whole wheat products, quinoa, brown rice, and oats.
- **Lean Proteins:** Canned beans, lentils, chickpeas, canned tuna, and low-sodium broth.
- **Healthy Fats:** Olive oil, nuts, seeds, and nut butters.
- **Low-Calorie Snacks**: Rice cakes, dried seaweed, and air-popped popcorn.

**Keep Your Fridge Fresh:** Store fresh, low-calorie ingredients that are easy to grab and use:
- **Fruits and Vegetables:** Stock a variety of fresh produce such as leafy greens, carrots, bell peppers, cucumbers, apples, and berries.
- **Lean Proteins**: Include eggs, chicken breast, turkey, tofu, and low-fat dairy products such as Greek yogurt and cottage cheese.
- **Prepared Items:** Have homemade sauces, dressings, and pre-portioned meals ready to go.

**Invest in Essential Tools and Resources:** Equipping your kitchen with the correct tools can make meal preparation quicker and more efficient:
- **Digital Food Scale:** Allows you to correctly measure portions while staying under your calorie restriction.
- **Measuring Cups and Spoons:** Essential for controlling serving sizes.
- **Meal Prep Containers:** Reusable containers for storing pre-portioned meals and snacks, making it simpler to access nutritious options when on the go.

- **Blender or Food Processor:** Useful for making smoothies, soups, sauces, and more.
- **Water Bottle:** Helps you monitor how much water you drink each day and keeps you hydrated throughout the day.

**Plan Your Weekly Meals and Prep in Advance:**
- **Meal Planning:** Dedicate a portion of your week to organize your meal plans. Choose what you'll eat for breakfast, lunch, dinner, and snacks to ensure it aligns with your 1200-calorie target.
- **Prep Ingredients in Batches:** Prepare ingredients like vegetables, fruits, lean proteins, and grains in advance to save time during the week.
- **Cook in Bulk:** Prepare larger portions of dishes that can be stored in the refrigerator or freezer, such as soups, stews, grilled chicken, or roasted vegetables.
- **Portion Out Meals:** Separate meals into individual servings with meal prep containers. This helps with portion control and ensures you stay within your calorie limit.
- **Label and Store Properly:** To ensure freshness, clearly mark your containers with the meal and the date.

> **Real-Life Example:** Mark, a father of two, found that meal prepping was a game-changer. " I used to be too busy to cook, so I would either miss meals or get takeout. But meal prepping on Sundays means I always have healthy options ready. It's helped me stay on track and save money."

## 3.2 MASTERING PORTION CONTROL AND HYDRATION

Portion control and hydration are essential components of the Dr. Now 1200-Calorie Diet Plan. Properly managing portion sizes ensures that you stay within your calorie limit while still feeling satisfied, and staying hydrated supports overall health and weight loss.

**Portion Control Strategies:**
- **Measure Your Food:** Use a digital food scale, measuring cups, and spoons to precisely measure your portions.
- **Use Smaller Plates and Bowls:** This trick will help you cut portion sizes while keeping you satisfied.
- **Follow the Plate Method:** Split your plate in half and put veggies on half of it. Put lean protein on the other quarter of your plate, and put whole grains or vegetables on the last quarter.

**Hydration Tips:**
- **Drink Water Before Meals:** Sip a glass of water to help you curb your appetite and prevent overindulgence.
- **Carry a Water Bottle:** Keep a water bottle on hand at all times to remind yourself to hydrate throughout the day.

- **Aim for at Least 8 Cups a Day:** Drinking at least 8 cups (64 ounces) of water daily helps support metabolism and digestion.
- **Avoid Caloric Beverages:** Avoid sugary drinks, sodas, and excessive alcohol, which add unnecessary calories without nutritional benefits. Instead, choose water, herbal infusions, or flavored water without added sugars.

> **Real-Life Example:** Lisa noticed that her portion sizes were creeping up, which was stalling her weight loss progress. She started using a smaller plate and noted, "I felt just as satisfied but was eating less. It's incredible how a simple modification can have a great impact!"

## 3.3 SMART GROCERY SHOPPING STRATEGIES

Shopping smart is key to staying on track with your diet while managing your budget. Here are some tips to help you make the most of your grocery trips:

**Make a Shopping List:** Plan your meals for the week and create a detailed shopping list based on your meal plan. Stick to the list to prevent impulsive purchases that might not support your objectives.

**Shop the Perimeter:** Pay attention to the grocery store's outside aisles, which are usually where you'll find fresh vegetables, dairy, lean meats, and whole grains.

**Look for Sales and Buy in Bulk:** Take advantage of sales, discounts, and bulk-buying opportunities for non-perishable items like grains, beans, and nuts. This can help you save money while stocking up on healthy essentials.

**Choose Seasonal and Frozen Produce:** Seasonal produce is frequently more reasonably priced, tastier, and fresher. Frozen fruits and vegetables are also a fantastic choice because they are typically more affordable and frozen at their optimal freshness, maintaining their nutrients.

**Read Food Labels:** For information on sodium, bad fats, and hidden sugars, always read the nutrition labels. Choose products that have less ingredients and no sugar or preservatives added.

**Be Flexible with Brands:** Don't be afraid to try generic or store brands; they are often cheaper and just as nutritious as name-brand products.

> **Real-Life Example:** Maria, who is on a tight budget, shares, "I started sticking to a shopping list and focusing on the perimeter of the store. It not only helped me eat healthier but also cut my grocery bill by 20%!"

### Conclusion: Equipping Yourself for Success

By combining these strategies—preparing your kitchen, mastering portion control and hydration, and shopping smart—you are setting yourself up for success on the Dr. Now 1200-Calorie Diet.

# CHAPTER 4: OVERCOMING COMMON CHALLENGES

Embarking on a weight loss journey comes with its hurdles, but mastering how to tackle them can make a big difference. This chapter addresses common hurdles such as cravings, emotional eating, social situations, and plateaus. By equipping yourself with practical strategies, you'll find yourself more equipped to maintain your path and reach your objectives.

## 4.1 HANDLING CRAVINGS AND EMOTIONAL EATING

Cravings and emotional eating are common barriers on the road to weight loss. Understanding their root causes and developing effective strategies to manage them can help you maintain control and continue progressing toward your goals.

**Identify Triggers:** Start by recognizing the situations, emotions, or environments that trigger your cravings or emotional eating. Is it stress, boredom, social gatherings, or certain times of the day? Keeping a journal to log your feelings and eating habits can help you pinpoint these triggers and understand when you're most vulnerable.

**Practice Mindful Eating:** Enjoy your meal at your own pace. When you eat, use all of your senses and relish every bite. This can lessen your propensity to eat mindlessly in reaction to emotions and help you feel more satiated with fewer servings.

Acknowledge your hunger cues—are you eating because you're hungry or because you're emotional?

**Find Healthy Alternatives:** When cravings hit, have healthier alternatives on hand that align with your 1200-calorie plan. If you want something sweet, have some fruit or a little dark chocolate. If you want something crunchy, try air-popped popcorn or sliced vegetables with a low-calorie dip.

**Engage in Stress-Relieving Activities:** Cravings are often triggered by stress or bad emotions. Try deep breathing, meditation, yoga, or a quick walk outside to help manage stress. Finding non-food coping mechanisms will help reduce emotional eating.

---

**Real-Life Example:** Jennifer found that her biggest cravings hit in the late afternoon when she was tired from work. By identifying this pattern, she started planning a healthy snack at that time—a small apple with a spoonful of almond butter. She also began taking a quick walk around the block to reset her mind. "It made a huge difference," she says. "I stopped reaching for junk food because I had a plan."

---

## 4.2 MANAGING SOCIAL SITUATIONS AND DINING OUT

Social situations and dining out can challenge even the most dedicated dieter. However, you may still enjoy these moments without sacrificing your objectives if you prepare ahead of time and make wise decisions.

**Plan Ahead:** Look over the menu or ask the host about the possibilities before heading to a social gathering or eating out. This enables you to avoid rash decisions and make well-informed ones. To help control your hunger, think about having a small, healthy whilstsnack before you leave.

**Choose Wisely:** Opt for lean protein options like grilled chicken or fish and go for steamed or roasted vegetables instead of fried or creamy sides. Avoid high-calorie dressings, sauces, and sugary beverages. If dining at a buffet, choose smaller portions and prioritize nutrient-dense foods.

**Practice Portion Control:** Eat in moderation and prevent overeating. If you have leftovers for another supper, think about sharing a dish with a friend or getting a take-out box.

To determine the right serving size, use visual cues such as comparing portion sizes to well-known items (for example, a tennis ball can help visualize the amount of pasta or fruit).

**Stay Hydrated:** Water consumption before, during, and after meals can help manage appetite and stop overeating. Carry a water bottle with you to remind yourself to stay hydrated.

**Communicate Your Needs:** Speak freely about your dietary choices or restrictions to friends, relatives, or staff members of a restaurant. Remember, your health and goals are a priority, and those around you should respect your choices.

**Focus on Socializing, Not Just the Food:** Remember that social gatherings are about more than simply eating; put your attention on mingling rather than just the cuisine. Take part in activities, strike up discussions, and enjoy the moment. If you take your mind off of the food, you can enjoy the event without feeling like you missed out.

---

**Real-Life Example:** Tom worried about an upcoming family reunion and the potential to overeat. He decided to review the restaurant's menu in advance and chose a healthy grilled fish dish. He also informed his family about his dietary goals, and they were supportive. At the event, he focused on catching up with relatives, and by sticking to his plan, he left feeling satisfied and proud of himself.

---

## 4.3 ADDRESSING NUTRITIONAL DEFICIENCIES SAFELY

A 1200-calorie diet can raise concerns about potential nutritional deficiencies, but with careful planning, you can ensure your body gets all the essential nutrients it needs.

**Focus on Foods Rich in Nutrients:** Make every calorie matter by selecting foods high in essential nutrients. Choose whole grains, fruits, veggies, lean proteins, and healthy fats. These foods supply the vitamins, minerals, and antioxidants your body needs to maintain general health.

**Consider Supplementation:** In certain cases, taking supplements may be necessary to achieve your nutritional requirements. Consult with a healthcare professional to determine if you require any specific supplements, such as multivitamins or omega-3 fatty acids.

**Monitor Your Intake:** Keep note of your daily food intake to ensure you are reaching your nutritional needs. Use a food diary or a mobile app to track your meals and snacks, and identify any potential nutrient gaps.

**Include a Variety of Foods:** Eating different foods can lower the chance of deficits. Try to have a colorful plate with different fruits, veggies, whole grains, and proteins for a good mix of nutrients.

**Consult a Registered Dietitian:** If you're unsure about how to meet your nutritional needs on a 1200-calorie diet, consider seeking guidance from a registered dietitian.

> **Real-Life Example:** Linda, worried about getting enough nutrients, consulted a dietitian who recommended adding more colorful vegetables to her diet and suggested a multivitamin. "I felt reassured knowing I was covering my bases," she says.

## 4.4 WHAT TO DO WHEN YOU HIT A PLATEAU

Weight reduction plateaus are common and can be discouraging, but they are an expected part of the process. Here is a step-by-step action plan to help you break through a plateau and continue making progress:

**Reevaluate Your Calorie Intake:** Take a closer look at your daily calorie intake and make sure you're still adhering to the 1200-calorie plan. Adjust portion sizes if needed and double-check for hidden calories in condiments, beverages, or snacks.

**Review Portion Sizes:** Ensure you're accurately measuring your food portions. Overestimating or underestimating portion sizes can impact your calorie intake and hinder progress.

**Consider Macronutrient Balance:** Adjust your macronutrient ratios if needed. For example, boosting protein intake might help maintain muscle mass and induce satiety, while limiting carbohydrates may aid in fat loss for some individuals.

**Fine-Tune Your Meal Plan:** If you're getting bored or dissatisfied with your meals, try new recipes or ingredients that fit within the plan's guidelines. Adding variety can help you stay motivated and committed.

**Increase Physical Activity:** Adding regular exercise to your routine can enhance your metabolic rate. Try to do moderate aerobic activity for at least two hours each week. Consider completing strength training exercises to increase your resting metabolic rate and build muscle.

**Mix Up Your Workouts:** Your body might have become accustomed to the routine if you've been performing the same exercises for a while. To keep your muscles and metabolism active, try a variety of workouts like yoga, swimming, or high-intensity interval training (HIIT).

**Seek Support:** If you're having trouble making changes, think about getting individualized counsel from a support group, a qualified dietician, or a healthcare professional.

**Stay Patient and Persistent:** Remember that weight loss is a gradual process, and plateaus are a normal part of that process. Persist in your goal-setting, have faith in the process, and keep making healthy choices.

> **Real-Life Example**: Emily hit a plateau after losing 15 pounds. By adding two days of strength training to her weekly routine and tweaking her meal plan to include more protein, she broke through the plateau and continued to lose weight steadily. "I learned that my body needed a little change to keep progressing," she shares.

## 4.5 CELEBRATING VICTORIES AND STAYING MOTIVATED

Celebrating your progress—both on and off the scale—is essential for maintaining motivation and positive momentum. Here's how to acknowledge your achievements and stay inspired:

### Recognize Non-Scale Victories

Celebrate all forms of progress, not just weight loss. Non-scale victories might include:

- Increased energy levels
- Improved sleep quality
- Enhanced mood and mental clarity
- Better-fitting clothes
- Reduced cravings
- Lowered blood pressure or cholesterol levels

These changes are important indicators of overall health and well-being, so take time to acknowledge them.

### Create Small Rewards for Milestones

When you hit a milestone, reward yourself with something other than food.
Here are some ideas:

- **Spa Day:** Book a massage, facial, or relaxing spa treatment.
- **New Workout Outfit:** Buy a new pair of leggings, sneakers, or fitness gear that makes you feel great.
- **Fun Outing:** Plan a day trip, a visit to a museum, or a movie night with friends.
- **Personal Development:** Choose a course, book, or workshop that you find exciting.
- **Hobby Supplies:** Purchase materials for a hobby you love, like painting, gardening, or crafting.

Rewards help reinforce your achievements and provide motivation to keep moving forward.

### Reflect on Your Progress Regularly

Take time to reflect on your trip and enjoy your accomplishments. Use setbacks as learning opportunities, and remember that growth is not always linear. Every step forward, however tiny, is a success.

### Remain Aware of Your "Why"

Remind yourself often of why you embarked on this quest.
Reflect on your goals and the positive changes you've experienced so far. It will be easier for you to remain motivated when you have a clear "why" in mind.

# CHAPTER 5: YOUR ESSENTIAL FOOD GUIDE FOR THE DR. NOW DIET

This chapter presents a straightforward guide to help you quickly identify which foods to embrace and which to avoid on the Dr. Now 1200-Calorie Diet. Use this as a quick guide for meal planning, shopping, and keeping up with your weight loss goals.

**Foods to Avoid**

These foods can derail your progress by adding unnecessary calories, sugars, unhealthy fats, and refined carbs. It's best to eliminate or limit them as much as possible:

- **Sugary Foods:** Candy, pastries, sugary cereals, ice cream
- **Refined Carbohydrates:** Pasta, white bread, crackers, bagels
- **High-Fat Foods:** Fried foods, fatty meats, full-fat dairy
- **Sugary Drinks and Alcohol:** Sodas, sweetened teas, beer, wine
- **Processed Foods:** Pre-packaged meals, processed meats, high-sodium snacks

**Foods to Choose**

Pay attention to these nutrient-dense foods that will help you lose weight and feel content and full:

- **Lean Proteins:** Chicken breast, fish, tofu, legumes, low-fat dairy
- **Low-Carb Vegetables:** Leafy greens, broccoli, zucchini, bell peppers
- **Whole Grains:** Quinoa, oats, brown rice, whole wheat products
- **Healthy Fats (in moderation):** Nuts, seeds, avocado, olive oil
- **Low-Calorie Snacks:** Fresh fruits, air-popped popcorn, raw veggies
- **Beverages:** Water, herbal teas, black coffee

**Conclusion: Keep It Simple and Smart**

By using this list, you can make quick, effective choices that align with the Dr. Now Diet. Focus on what nourishes your body and avoid foods that may hamper your progress.

# CHAPTER 6: BREAKFAST RECIPES

## SPINACH AND MUSHROOM OMELETTE

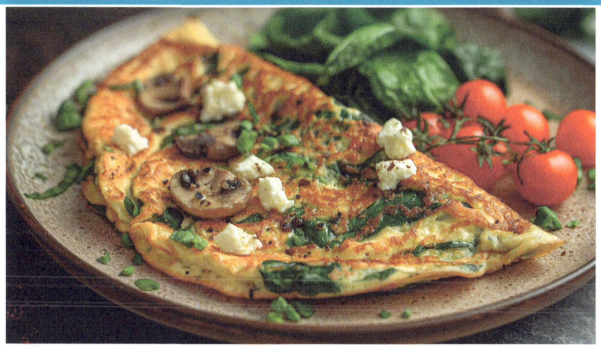

**PREP TIME:** 10 min

**COOK TIME:** 10 min

**COOKING METHOD:** Stovetop

**Servings:** 2

**Ingredients:**

- 4 large eggs
- 1 cup spinach, chopped
- 1/2 cup mushrooms, sliced
- 1/4 cup **reduced-fat** cheddar cheese
- 1 teaspoon olive oil
- Salt and pepper to taste

**Steps:**

1. In a mixing bowl, beat the eggs until thoroughly blended.
2. Heat the olive oil in a nonstick pan over medium heat.
3. Add the mushrooms and sauté until they release their moisture.
4. Add the spinach and cook until wilted.
5. Pour the beaten eggs into the skillet and cook until the edges start to set.
6. Sprinkle the reduced-fat cheddar cheese over the omelette.
7. Using a spatula, fold the omelette in half, then cook for one more minute.
8. Add salt and pepper to taste.

**Tips:**

- For balanced breakfast, serve with fresh fruit on the side. Add other vegetables or herbs for customization.

**Nutritional Values:**

Calories: 200, Fat: 12g, Carbs: 3g, Protein: 16g, Sugar: 1g

# GREEK YOGURT PARFAIT

**PREP TIME:** 10 min
**COOK TIME:** 0 min
**COOKING METHOD:** No cooking required
**Servings:** 1
**Ingredients:**

- 1 cup plain **non-fat** Greek yogurt
- 1/2 cup mixed berries (strawberries, blueberries, raspberries)
- 2 tablespoons **unsweetened oats** or chopped nuts
- 1 teaspoon honey

**Steps:**

1. In a glass or bowl, layer half of the Greek yogurt.
2. Place half of the mixed berries on top of the yogurt.
3. Sprinkle half of the oats or nuts over the berries.
4. Continue layering with the remaining ingredients.
5. Drizzle honey over the top of the parfait.

**Tips:**

- You can add nuts or seeds for added crunch and flavor.
- Use flavored Greek yogurt (without added sugars) for variety.

**Nutritional Values:**
Calories: 240, Fat: 5g, Carbs: 30g, Protein: 20g, Sugar: 10g

# QUINOA BREAKFAST BOWL

**PREP TIME:** 5 min
**COOK TIME:** 15 min
**COOKING METHOD:** Stovetop

- **Servings:** 2

**Ingredients:**

- 1 cup cooked quinoa
- 1/2 cup **unsweetened and unflavored** almond milk
- 1/4 cup of almonds, chopped
- 1/4 cup **unsweetened** dried cranberries or fresh fruit
- 1/2 teaspoon cinnamon

**Steps:**

1. In a saucepan, heat the cooked quinoa and almond milk over medium heat.
2. Stir in the chopped almonds, unsweetened cranberries, and cinnamon.
3. Cook until heated through and the flavors are well combined.
4. Divide the quinoa mixture into bowls and serve.

**Tips:**

- Add fresh fruits or other toppings for variety.
- Use any type of milk or milk alternative based on preference.

**Nutritional Values:**
Calories: 280, Fat: 8g, Carbs: 40g, Protein: 10g, Sugar: 8g

# VEGETABLE FRITTATA

**PREP TIME:** 10 min
**COOK TIME:** 20 min
**COOKING METHOD:** Stovetop and Oven
**Servings:** 4

**Ingredients:**

- 6 large eggs
- 1/2 cup chopped bell peppers
- 1/2 cup chopped onions
- 1/2 cup chopped zucchini
- 1/4 cup **reduced-fat** cheddar cheese
- 1 teaspoon olive oil
- Salt and pepper to taste

**Steps:**

1. Preheat the oven to 375°F (190°C).
2. Beat the eggs in a basin until they are thoroughly combined.
3. Heat olive oil in an oven-safe skillet over medium heat.
4. Add the chopped bell peppers, onions, and zucchini to the skillet and sauté until tender.
5. Pour the beaten eggs over the sautéed vegetables in the skillet.
6. Sprinkle the reduced-fat cheddar cheese over the eggs and vegetables.
7. Add salt and pepper according to taste.
8. Move the skillet to the preheated oven and bake till the frittata is set and golden on top 15 to 20 minutes.
9. Remove the dish from the oven and allow it to chill before serving.

**Tips:**

- Add other vegetables or herbs to taste. Serve with a side salad.

**Nutritional Values:**

Calories: 180, Fat: 10g, Carbs: 6g, Protein: 12g, Sugar: 3g

## TOMATO AND AVOCADO BREAKFAST SALAD

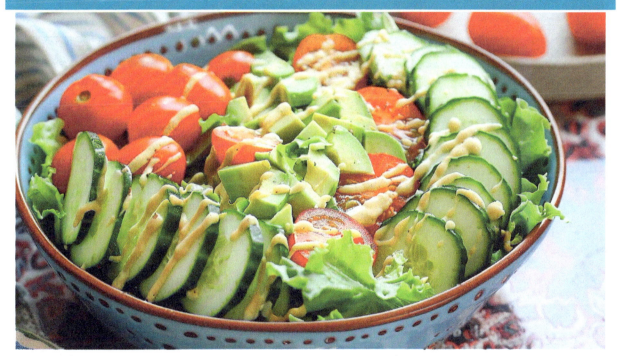

**PREP TIME:** 10 min
**COOK TIME:** None
**COOKING METHOD:** No cooking required
**Servings:** 2
**Ingredients:**

- 1 cup cherry tomatoes, halved
- 1/2 avocado, diced
- 1/4 cup diced cucumber
- 1 tablespoon lemon juice
- 1 tablespoon chopped fresh parsley
- Salt and pepper to taste

**Steps:**

1. In a bowl, combine the tomatoes, avocado, cucumber, lemon juice, and parsley.
2. Add salt and pepper and gently toss to combine.

**Tips:**

Serve with a boiled egg or whole grain toast for added protein and fiber.

**Nutritional Values:**

Calories: 120, Fat: 9g, Carbs: 9g, Protein: 2g, Sugar: 3g

## COTTAGE CHEESE AND BERRY BOWL

**PREP TIME:** 5 min

**COOK TIME:** None

**COOKING METHOD:** No cooking required

**Servings:** 1

**Ingredients:**

- 1 cup low-fat cottage cheese
- 1/2 cup mixed berries (strawberries, blueberries, raspberries)
- 1 tablespoon chopped almonds
- 1/2 teaspoon honey (optional)

**Steps:**

1. Layer cottage cheese and mixed berries in a bowl.
2. Add chopped almonds and honey if preferred.

**Tips:**

- Use different fruits like peaches or pineapple for variety.

**Nutritional Values:**

Calories: 160, Fat: 5g, Carbs: 15g, Protein: 20g, Sugar: 8g

## SWEET POTATO HASH

**PREP TIME:** 10 min

**COOK TIME:** 20 min

**COOKING METHOD:** Stovetop

**Servings:** 2

**Ingredients:**

- 1 large sweet potato, peeled and diced
- 1/2 cup diced bell peppers
- 1/2 cup diced onions
- 1 teaspoon olive oil
- 1/2 teaspoon paprika
- 1/4 teaspoon garlic powder
- Salt and pepper to taste

**Steps:**

1. In a large skillet, heat olive oil over medium heat.
2. Add the diced sweet potato, bell peppers, and onions to the skillet.
3. Sprinkle paprika, garlic powder, salt, and pepper over the vegetables.
4. Sauté until the sweet potato is cooked through and slightly crispy.
5. Remove from heat and serve hot.

**Tips:**

- For extra taste top with a fried egg or avocado slices Feel free to add other vegetables or spices.

**Nutritional Values:**

Calories: 210, Fat: 8g, Carbs: 30g, Protein: 3g, Sugar: 6g

# TURKEY AND VEGGIE BREAKFAST WRAP

**PREP TIME:** 5 min

**COOK TIME:** 5 min

**COOKING METHOD:** Stovetop

**Servings:** 1

**Ingredients:**

- 1 whole wheat tortilla
- 2 slices lean turkey breast
- 1/4 cup sliced bell peppers
- 1/4 cup baby spinach
- 1 tablespoon hummus

**Steps:**

1. Warm the tortilla in a skillet over medium heat for 1-2 minutes.
2. Spread hummus on the tortilla, then layer with turkey, bell peppers, and spinach.
3. Roll up the tortilla tightly and serve.

**Tips:**

- Wrap in foil for an easy on-the-go breakfast.

**Nutritional Values:**

Calories: 180, Fat: 5g, Carbs: 20g, Protein: 15g, Sugar: 2g

# APPLE CINNAMON OATMEAL

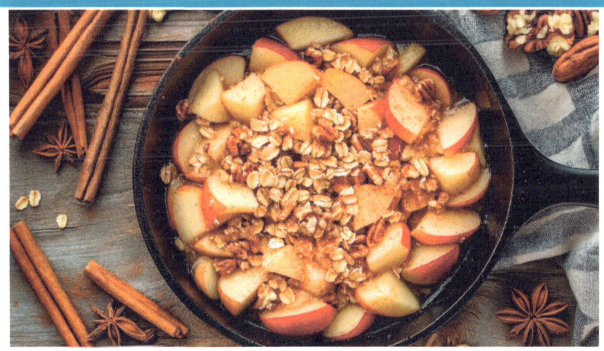

**PREP TIME:** 5 min

**COOK TIME:** 10 min

**COOKING METHOD:** Stovetop

**Servings:** 1

**Ingredients:**

- 1/2 cup rolled oats
- 1 cup water or unsweetened almond milk
- 1/2 apple, diced
- 1/2 teaspoon ground cinnamon
- 1 tablespoon chopped walnuts
- 1/2 teaspoon vanilla extract

**Steps:**

1. In a saucepan, bring the water or almond milk to a boil.
2. Add cinnamon, apple chunks, rolled oats, and vanilla essence.

3. Reduce heat and simmer until oats are cooked and mixture thickens.
4. Top with chopped walnuts before serving.

**Tips:**
- Add a sprinkle of flax seeds or chia seeds for extra nutrition.

**Nutritional Values:**

Calories: 200, Fat: 7g, Carbs: 33g, Protein: 5g, Sugar: 10g

## SCRAMBLED EGG WHITES WITH VEGGIES

**PREP TIME:** 5 min
**COOK TIME:** 5 min
**COOKING METHOD:** Stovetop
Servings: 2
**Ingredients:**
- 6 egg whites
- 1/2 cup chopped spinach
- 1/4 cup diced tomatoes
- 1/4 cup diced bell peppers
- 1/4 cup diced onions
- 1 tablespoon olive oil
- Salt and pepper to taste

**Steps:**
- In a bowl, whisk the egg whites until foamy.
- Heat olive oil in a non-stick skillet over medium heat.
- Add the onions, bell peppers, and tomatoes, sautéing until softened.
- Add the spinach and sauté till wilted.
- Pour in the egg whites and scramble gently until fully cooked.
- Add salt and pepper.

**Tips:**
- Serve with a side of whole wheat toast or fresh fruit.

**Nutritional Values:**

Calories: 100, Fat: 5g, Carbs: 5g, Protein: 12g, Sugar: 2g

## ALMOND BUTTER BANANA TOAST

**PREP TIME:** 5 min
**COOK TIME:** None
**COOKING METHOD:** No cooking required
Servings: 1
**Ingredients:**
- 1 slice whole wheat bread, toasted
- 1 tablespoon almond butter
- 1/2 small banana, sliced
- 1/4 teaspoon ground cinnamon

**Steps:**
1. Spread almond butter evenly on the toasted bread.
2. Arrange the banana slices on top and sprinkle with cinnamon.

**Tips:**
- Add chia seeds or flax seeds for extra fiber.

**Nutritional Values:**

Calories: 220, Fat: 9g, Carbs: 28g, Protein: 6g, Sugar: 10g

# CHIA PUDDING

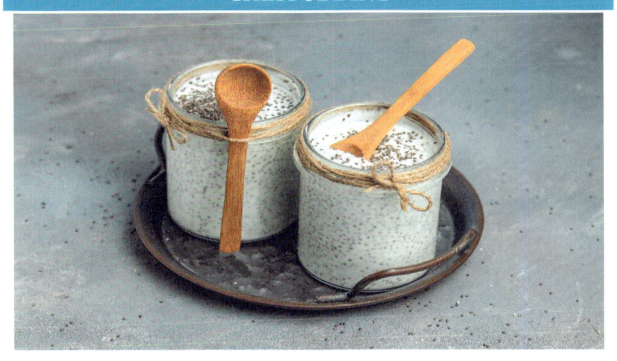

**PREP TIME:** 5 min

**COOK TIME:** 4 hours (chilling time)

**COOKING METHOD:** No cooking required

**Servings:** 2

**Ingredients:**

- 1/4 cup chia seeds
- 1 cup unsweetened almond milk
- 1/4 teaspoon vanilla extract

**Steps:**

1. Mix the almond milk, vanilla essence, and chia seeds in a basin or container.
2. Stir well to evenly distribute chia seeds.
3. Place in the refrigerator for at least 4 hours, or overnight, until the mixture has thickened.
4. Before serving, stir and distribute chia pudding into bowls or glasses.

**Tips:**

- Top with fresh fruits or nuts for added flavor.
- Try out a variety of flavors such as cocoa powder or matcha.

**Nutritional Values:**

Calories: 130, Fat: 7g, Carbs: 12g, Protein: 4g, Sugar: 2g

# ZUCCHINI AND EGG MUFFINS

**PREP TIME:** 10 min

**COOK TIME:** 20 min

**COOKING METHOD:** Oven

**Servings:** 4

**Ingredients:**

- 4 large eggs
- 1/2 cup grated zucchini
- 1/4 cup chopped spinach
- 1/4 cup diced bell peppers
- 1/4 cup low-fat feta cheese
- Salt and pepper to taste

**Steps:**

1. Preheat the oven to 375°F (190°C).
2. In a bowl, beat the eggs and add zucchini, spinach, bell peppers, and feta cheese.
3. Season with salt and pepper.
4. Pour the mixture into a muffin tray that has been oiled or lined with paper cups.
5. Bake for 15-20 minutes, or until the muffins are set.

**Tips:**

- Store in the refrigerator for quick grab-and-go breakfasts throughout the week.

**Nutritional Values:**

Calories: 100, Fat: 5g, Carbs: 4g, Protein: 10g, Sugar: 1g

## POACHED EGGS WITH ASPARAGUS

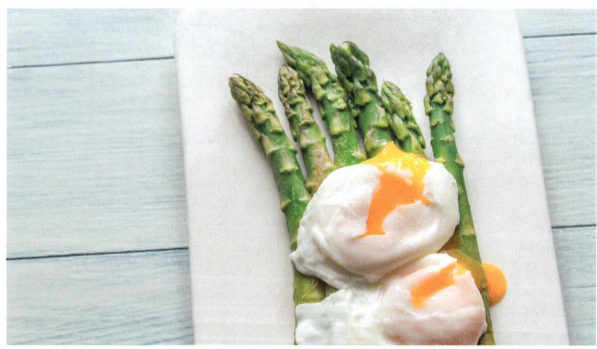

**PREP TIME:** 5 min
**COOK TIME:** 10 min
**COOKING METHOD:** Stovetop
**Servings:** 2
**Ingredients:**

- 4 large eggs
- 1/2 bunch asparagus, trimmed
- 1 tablespoon vinegar
- Salt and pepper to taste

**Steps:**

1. Bring a saucepan of water to a low heat, then add vinegar.
2. Place each egg in a cup and gently slip it into simmering water. Poach for 3–4 minutes.
3. Meanwhile, steam or boil the asparagus until tender.
4. Serve the poached eggs over the asparagus and season with salt and pepper.

**Tips:**

- Pair with a slice of whole grain toast for added fiber.

**Nutritional Values:**

Calories: 150, Fat: 10g, Carbs: 4g, Protein: 12g, Sugar: 2g

# CHAPTER 7: MAIN DISHES

## 7.1 POULTRY: LEAN CHICKEN & TURKEY

### GRILLED CHICKEN SALAD

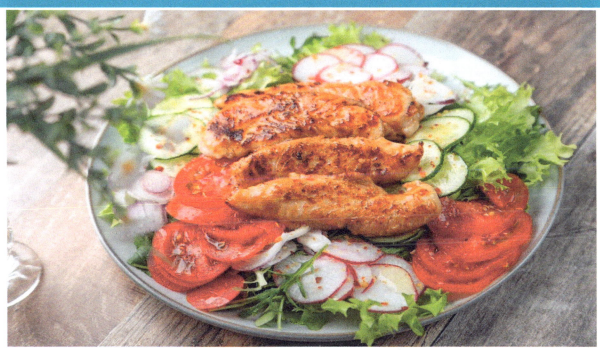

**PREP TIME:** 10 min
**COOK TIME:** 10 min
**COOKING METHOD:** Grilling
**Servings:** 2
**Ingredients:**

- 2 boneless, skinless chicken breasts
- 4 cups mixed greens (lettuce, spinach, arugula)
- 1/2 cup cherry tomatoes, halved
- 1/4 cucumber, sliced
- 1/4 cup shredded carrots
- 1 tablespoon olive oil
- 1 tablespoon lemon juice
- Salt and pepper to taste

**Steps:**

1. Season the chicken breasts with salt and pepper.
2. Grill the chicken over medium heat for approximately 5-6 minutes on each side until it is thoroughly cooked.
3. Before slicing, let the chicken a few minutes to rest.
4. In a large bowl, mix together the mixed greens, cherry tomatoes, cucumber, and shredded carrots.
5. Add sliced grilled chicken on top.
6. Before serving, drizzle the salad with olive oil and lemon juice.

**Tips:**

- Add a handful of sliced almonds or a sprinkle of flaxseed for extra crunch and nutrition.

**Nutritional Values:**

Calories: 250, Fat: 10g, Carbs: 12g, Protein: 30g, Sugar: 5g

## TURKEY LETTUCE WRAPS

**PREP TIME:** 10 min

**COOK TIME:** 10 min

**COOKING METHOD:** Stovetop

**Servings:** 4

**Ingredients:**

- 1 pound lean ground turkey
- 1/2 onion, diced
- 2 cloves garlic, minced
- 1/2 red bell pepper, diced
- 1/2 cup shredded carrots
- 1 tablespoon low-sodium soy sauce
- 1 tablespoon hoisin sauce (optional)
- 1 teaspoon olive oil
- Big lettuce leaves (like romaine or butter lettuce) for wrapping
- Salt and pepper to taste

**Steps:**

1. Warm olive oil in a skillet set to medium heat.
2. Sauté onion and garlic until fragrant.
3. Add ground turkey, continue cooking until no longer pink.
4. Stir in bell pepper, carrots, soy sauce, and hoisin sauce.
5. Continue cooking for an additional 3-5 minutes until the vegetables become tender.
6. Spoon the mixture into large lettuce leaves and wrap.

**Tips:**

- Add a dash of sriracha or red pepper flakes for extra spice.

**Nutritional Values:**

Calories: 210, Fat: 9g, Carbs: 7g, Protein: 28g, Sugar: 3g

## GRILLED CHICKEN AND VEGETABLE SKEWERS

**PREP TIME:** 15 min

**COOK TIME:** 10 min

**COOKING METHOD:** Grill

**Servings:** 2

**Ingredients:**

- 2 chicken breasts, cubed
- 1 zucchini, sliced
- 1 red onion, cut into wedges
- 1 red bell pepper, diced
- 1 tablespoon olive oil
- 1 teaspoon lemon juice
- Salt and pepper to taste

**Steps:**

1. Set the grill's temperature to medium-high.
2. Thread veggies and chicken onto skewers.
3. Brush with olive oil and lemon juice, and season with salt and pepper.
4. Grill for 8-10 minutes, turning occasionally, until chicken is well done.

**Tips:**

- Serve with a side of quinoa or a mixed green salad.

**Nutritional Values:**

Calories: 250, Fat: 9g, Carbs: 10g, Protein: 36g, Sugar: 4g

# TURKEY AND SPINACH STUFFED PEPPERS

**PREP TIME:** 15 min
**COOK TIME:** 30 min
**COOKING METHOD:** Oven
**Servings:** 4
**Ingredients:**

- 4 bell peppers, halved and seeded
- 1/2 pound ground turkey
- 2 cups spinach, chopped
- 1/2 cup cooked brown rice
- 1/4 cup diced tomatoes
- 1 tablespoon olive oil
- Salt and pepper to taste

**Steps:**

1. Begin by setting your oven to a temperature of 375°F (190°C).
2. In a skillet, warm olive oil over medium heat and sauté ground turkey until it turns a lovely brown.
3. Incorporate spinach, prepared rice, and chopped tomatoes into the skillet, and sauté for 5 minutes.
4. Stuff the halves of the bell peppers with the turkey mixture.
5. Arrange in a baking dish and cook for 25-30 minutes until the peppers are soft.

**Tips:**

- Top with a sprinkle of low-fat cheese if desired.

**Nutritional Values:**

Calories: 200, Fat: 8g, Carbs: 14g, Protein: 18g, Sugar: 3g

# ZUCCHINI NOODLES WITH TURKEY MEATBALLS

**PREP TIME:** 15 min
**COOK TIME:** 20 min
**COOKING METHOD:** Stovetop
**Servings:** 3
**Ingredients:**

- 2 medium zucchinis, spiralized into noodles
- 1/2 pound lean ground turkey
- 1/4 cup breadcrumbs (whole wheat or gluten-free)
- 1 egg
- 2 tablespoons Parmesan cheese, grated
- 2 cups marinara sauce (no added sugar)
- 1 tablespoon olive oil
- 1/2 teaspoon Italian seasoning
- Salt and pepper to taste

**Steps:**

1. In a bowl, mix ground turkey, breadcrumbs, egg, Parmesan cheese, Italian seasoning, salt, and pepper.
2. Form into small meatballs.
3. Warm olive oil in a skillet set to medium heat and sear the meatballs until they are golden brown on all sides.
4. Add marinara sauce to the skillet and let the meatballs cook for 10 to 15 minutes, or until they are fully cooked.
5. In another pan, gently cook the zucchini noodles for 2-3 minutes.
6. Serve meatballs and sauce over zucchini noodles.

**Tips:**
- Garnish with fresh basil or parsley.

**Nutritional Values:**
Calories: 280, Fat: 15g, Carbs: 14g, Protein: 25g, Sugar: 5g

## SPINACH AND FETA STUFFED CHICKEN BREAST

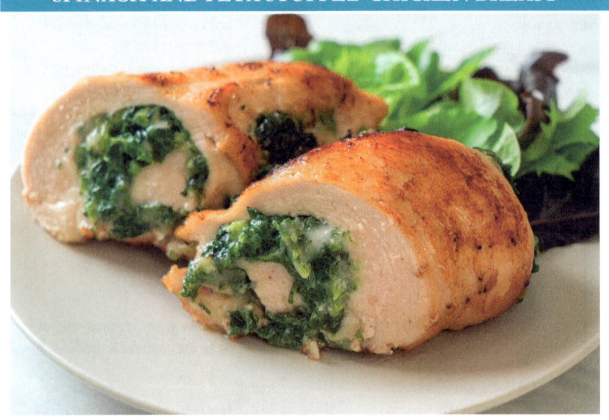

**PREP TIME:** 10 min
**COOK TIME:** 25 min
**COOKING METHOD:** Oven
**Servings:** 2
**Ingredients:**
- 2 boneless, skinless chicken breasts
- 1/2 cup spinach, chopped
- 1/4 cup feta cheese, crumbled
- 1 tablespoon olive oil
- Salt and pepper to taste

**Steps:**
1. Preheat the oven to 375°F (190°C).
2. Cut a pocket into each chicken breast and stuff with spinach and feta cheese.
3. Season with salt and pepper.
4. Warm olive oil in an oven-safe skillet and sear the chicken breasts on each side until they are golden.
5. Place the skillet to the oven and bake for 20-25 minutes, or until the chicken is completely cooked through.

**Tips:**
- Pair with steamed vegetables or a side salad.

**Nutritional Values:**
Calories: 280, Fat: 12g, Carbs: 2g, Protein: 38g, Sugar: 0g

# GRILLED LEMON HERB CHICKEN

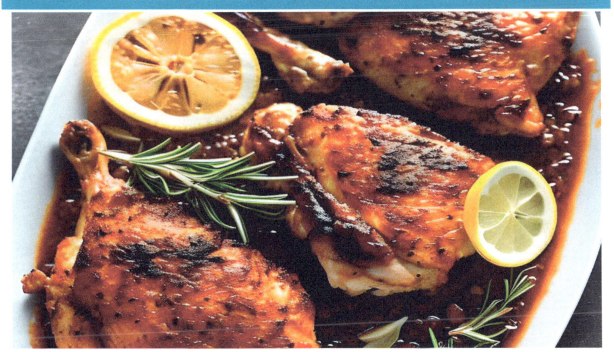

**PREP TIME:** 10 min

**COOK TIME:** 15 min

**COOKING METHOD:** Grill or Stovetop

**Servings:** 2

**Ingredients:**

- 2 chicken breasts without bones or skin
- 1 lemon, juiced
- 2 garlic cloves, minced
- 1 tablespoon olive oil
- 1 teaspoon dried oregano
- 1/2 teaspoon black pepper
- 1/4 teaspoon salt

**Steps:**

1. In a small bowl, combine lemon juice, minced garlic, olive oil, oregano, salt, and pepper.
2. Marinate the chicken breasts in this mixture for at least 30 minutes.
3. Preheat the grill or stovetop pan over medium heat.
4. Grill the chicken for about 6-7 minutes on each side until cooked through.
5. Serve hot with a side of steamed vegetables.

**Tips:**

- For added flavor, marinate the chicken for a few hours or overnight.
- Pair with a salad for a complete meal.

**Nutritional Values:**

Calories: 220, Fat: 9g, Carbs: 2g, Protein: 30g, Sugar: 0g

# TURKEY AND SPINACH MEATBALLS

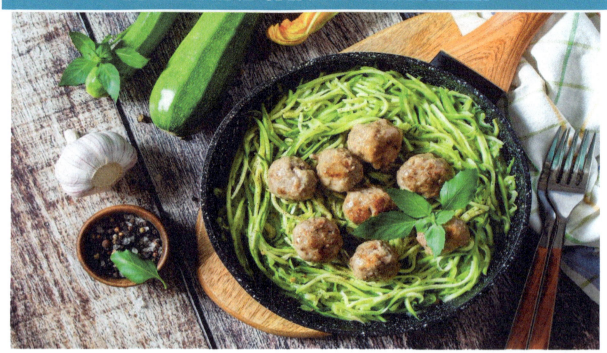

**PREP TIME:** 15 min

**COOK TIME:** 20 min

**COOKING METHOD:** Oven

**Servings:** 4

**Ingredients:**

- 1 lb lean ground turkey
- 1 cup fresh spinach, chopped
- 1/4 cup whole wheat breadcrumbs
- 1 egg
- 2 garlic cloves, minced
- 1 tablespoon olive oil
- 1 teaspoon dried oregano
- Salt and pepper to taste

**Steps:**

1. Preheat oven to 375°F (190°C).
2. In a bowl, combine ground turkey, spinach, breadcrumbs, egg, minced garlic, oregano, salt, and pepper.
3. Form mixture into small meatballs and place them on a baking sheet.
4. Drizzle with olive oil and bake for 18-20 minutes or until cooked through.
5. Serve hot with marinara sauce or a side of steamed vegetables.

**Tips:**

- Make extra meatballs and freeze for a quick meal later.
- Serve over zucchini noodles for a low-carb option.

**Nutritional Values:**

Calories: 200, Fat: 10g, Carbs: 5g, Protein: 25g, Sugar: 1g

## BAKED CHICKEN WITH CAULIFLOWER MASH

**PREP TIME:** 15 min
**COOK TIME:** 30 min
**COOKING METHOD:** Oven
**Servings:** 2
**Ingredients:**

- 2 boneless, skinless chicken breasts
- 1 head cauliflower, chopped into florets
- 1/4 cup low-fat milk
- 1 tablespoon olive oil
- 1 teaspoon garlic powder
- Salt and pepper to taste

**Steps:**

1. Preheat oven to 375°F (190°C).
2. Season chicken breasts with garlic powder, salt, and pepper.
3. Bake chicken for 25-30 minutes until cooked through.
4. While chicken bakes, steam cauliflower until tender.
5. Blend cauliflower with milk, olive oil, salt, and pepper until smooth.
6. Serve chicken with cauliflower mash.

**Tips:**

- Garnish the mash with chopped herbs for added flavor.
- Substitute chicken with fish or turkey for variation.

**Nutritional Values:**

Calories: 230, Fat: 9g, Carbs: 12g, Protein: 28g, Sugar: 3g

## TURKEY CHILI

**PREP TIME:** 15 min
**COOK TIME:** 40 min
**COOKING METHOD:** Stovetop
**Servings:** 4
**Ingredients:**

- 1 lb lean ground turkey
- 1 cup diced tomatoes
- 1/2 cup kidney beans, drained
- 1/2 cup black beans, drained
- 1/2 cup chopped onions
- 1/2 cup chopped bell peppers
- 1 tablespoon olive oil
- 2 garlic cloves, minced
- 1 teaspoon chili powder
- 1/2 teaspoon cumin
- Salt and pepper to taste

**Steps:**

1. Heat olive oil in a large pot over medium heat.
2. Add onions, garlic, and bell peppers; sauté until softened.
3. Add ground turkey, chili powder, cumin, salt, and pepper; cook until browned.
4. Stir in tomatoes and beans, bring to a boil, then reduce heat and simmer for 30 minutes.
5. Serve hot with a sprinkle of fresh herbs.

**Tips:**

- Make extra and freeze portions for a quick meal later.
- Top with a dollop of Greek yogurt for a creamy texture.

**Nutritional Values:**

Calories: 250, Fat: 8g, Carbs: 20g, Protein: 26g, Sugar: 5g

## CHICKEN AND VEGETABLE SKEWERS

**PREP TIME:** 15 min
**COOK TIME:** 15 min
**COOKING METHOD:** Grill
**Servings:** 4
**Ingredients:**

- 2 boneless, skinless chicken breasts, cut into cubes
- 1 cup bell peppers, cut into squares
- 1/2 cup zucchini, sliced
- 1/2 cup cherry tomatoes
- 1 tablespoon olive oil
- 1 tablespoon lemon juice
- 1 teaspoon dried oregano
- Salt and pepper to taste

**Steps:**

1. Preheat the grill to medium heat.
2. In a bowl, mix olive oil, lemon juice, oregano, salt, and pepper.
3. Thread chicken, bell peppers, zucchini, and cherry tomatoes onto skewers.
4. Brush the skewers with the marinade mixture.
5. Grill for 10-15 minutes, turning occasionally until chicken is cooked through.
6. Serve hot.

**Tips:**

- Soak wooden skewers in water for 30 minutes before grilling to prevent burning.
- Serve with a side of tzatziki sauce for added flavor.

**Nutritional Values:**

Calories: 180, Fat: 6g, Carbs: 5g, Protein: 28g, Sugar: 2g

## SPINACH AND MUSHROOM STUFFED CHICKEN BREAST

**PREP TIME:** 15 min
**COOK TIME:** 30 min
**COOKING METHOD:** Oven
**Servings:** 2
**Ingredients:**

- 2 chicken breasts
- 1 cup spinach, chopped
- 1/2 cup mushrooms, sliced
- 1/4 cup low-fat mozzarella cheese, shredded
- 1 tablespoon olive oil
- 1 garlic clove, minced
- Salt and pepper to taste

**Steps:**

1. Preheat oven to 375°F (190°C).
2. In a skillet, heat olive oil; sauté garlic, spinach, and mushrooms until wilted.
3. Slice chicken breasts lengthwise to create a pocket.
4. Stuff each chicken breast with the spinach and mushroom mixture and secure with toothpicks.
5. Place in a baking dish and bake for 25-30 minutes until cooked through.
6. Serve hot.

**Tips:**

- Use a meat thermometer to ensure the chicken is cooked to an internal temperature of 165°F (74°C).
- Serve with a side of roasted vegetables or a salad.

**Nutritional Values:**

Calories: 393, Fat: 15.5g, Carbs: 2.5g, Protein: 57.5g, Sugar: 0.6g

## LEMON GARLIC SHRIMP PASTA

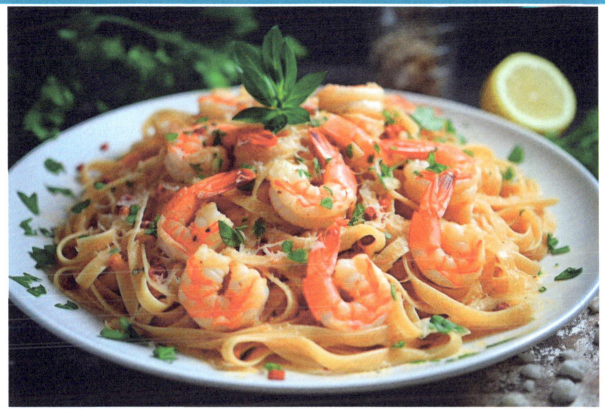

**PREP TIME:** 10 min
**COOK TIME:** 15 min
**COOKING METHOD:** Stovetop
**Servings:** 2

**Ingredients:**

- 4 ounces whole wheat pasta
- 1/2 pound shrimp, stripped of its shells
- 2 minced cloves of garlic.
- 1 tablespoon lemon juice
- 1 tablespoon olive oil
- 1/4 cup parsley, chopped
- Salt and pepper to taste

**Steps:**

1. Cook the pasta by following the directions on the package.
2. Heat olive oil in a skillet over medium heat, add garlic and sauté until fragrant.
3. Add shrimp and cook until pink, about 2-3 minutes per side.
4. Toss shrimp with cooked pasta, lemon juice, and parsley.
5. Add a sprinkle of salt and a dash of pepper before serving.

**Tips:**

- Add steamed broccoli or spinach for extra vegetables.

**Nutritional Values:**

Calories: 340, Fat: 10g, Carbs: 45g, Protein: 28g, Sugar: 3g

## TUNA AND WHITE BEAN SALAD

**PREP TIME:** 10 min

**COOK TIME:** 0 min

**COOKING METHOD:** No cooking required

**Servings:** 2

**Ingredients:**

- 1 can tuna in water, drained
- 1 cup white beans, rinsed and drained
- 1/2 red onion, finely chopped
- 1/4 cup fresh parsley, chopped
- 1 tablespoon lemon juice
- 1 tablespoon olive oil
- Salt and pepper to taste

**Steps:**

1. In a bowl, mix tuna, white beans, red onion, and parsley.
2. Drizzle with lemon juice and olive oil.
3. Season with salt and pepper and toss to combine.

**Tips:**

- Serve on whole wheat toast or alongside a green salad.

**Nutritional Values:**

Calories: 250, Fat: 12g, Carbs: 20g, Protein: 24g, Sugar: 2g

## SHRIMP AND AVOCADO SALAD

**PREP TIME:** 10 min

**COOK TIME:** 5 min

**COOKING METHOD:** Stovetop

**Servings:** 2

**Ingredients:**

- 1/2 pound shrimp, peeled and deveined
- 1 avocado, diced
- 1/2 cup cherry tomatoes, halved
- 2 cups mixed greens
- 1 tablespoon olive oil
- 1 tablespoon lemon juice
- Salt and pepper to taste

**Steps:**

1. Heat the olive oil in a pan over medium heat.
2. Cook shrimp for 2-3 minutes on each side until they turn pink and opaque.
3. In a bowl, combine mixed greens, avocado, cherry tomatoes, and cooked shrimp.
4. Drizzle with lemon juice, and season with salt and pepper.

**Tips:**

- Garnish with fresh cilantro or parsley for added flavor.

**Nutritional Values:**

Calories: 290, Fat: 18g, Carbs: 10g, Protein: 22g, Sugar: 3g

# BAKED COD WITH LEMON AND HERBS

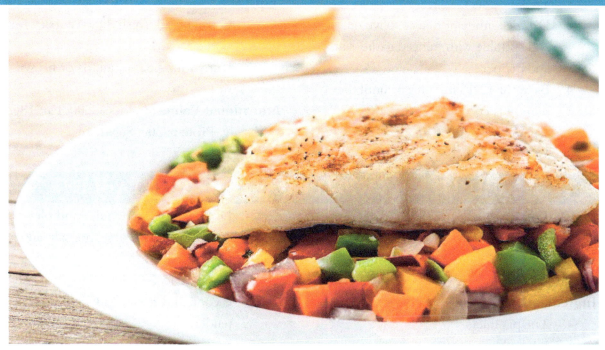

**PREP TIME:** 10 min

**COOK TIME:** 15 min

**COOKING METHOD:** Oven

**Servings:** 2

**Ingredients:**

- 2 cod fillets
- 1 lemon, sliced
- 2 garlic cloves, minced
- 1 tablespoon olive oil
- 1 teaspoon dried dill
- Salt and pepper to taste

**Steps:**

1. Preheat oven to 400°F (200°C).
2. Place cod fillets in a baking dish and drizzle with olive oil.
3. Sprinkle with minced garlic, dill, salt, and pepper.
4. Arrange lemon slices on top of the fillets.
5. Bake for 12-15 minutes or until fish is flaky and cooked through.
6. Serve with a side of steamed vegetables.

**Tips:**

- Use fresh herbs for a more robust flavor.
- Pair with a quinoa salad for a balanced meal.

**Nutritional Values:** Calories: 160, Fat: 6g, Carbs: 2g, Protein: 28g, Sugar: 0g

# SALMON WITH ASPARAGUS

**PREP TIME:** 10 min

**COOK TIME:** 15 min

**COOKING METHOD:** Oven

**Servings:** 2

**Ingredients:**

- 2 salmon fillets
- 1 bunch of asparagus, trimmed
- 2 tablespoons lemon juice
- 1 tablespoon olive oil
- 2 garlic cloves, minced
- Salt and pepper to taste

**Steps:**

1. Preheat oven to 400°F (200°C).

2. Place salmon fillets and asparagus on a baking sheet.
3. Drizzle with lemon juice, olive oil, and sprinkle with minced garlic, salt, and pepper.
4. Bake for 12-15 minutes or until the salmon is cooked through and asparagus is tender.

5. Serve hot.

**Tips:**

- Garnish with fresh dill or parsley for added flavor.
- Pair with a side of quinoa or brown rice.

**Nutritional Values:** Calories: 300, Fat: 18g, Carbs: 4g, Protein: 30g, Sugar: 1g

## BAKED TILAPIA WITH ROASTED VEGETABLES

**PREP TIME:** 10 min
**COOK TIME:** 20 min
**COOKING METHOD:** Oven
**Servings:** 2
**Ingredients:**

- 2 tilapia fillets
- 1 cup cherry tomatoes
- 1 cup zucchini, sliced
- 1/2 cup sliced red onion
- 2 tablespoons lemon juice
- 1 tablespoon olive oil
- 1 teaspoon dried oregano
- Salt and pepper to taste

**Steps:**

1. Preheat oven to 375°F (190°C).
2. Place tilapia fillets, cherry tomatoes, zucchini, and onions on a baking sheet.

3. Drizzle with lemon juice and olive oil; sprinkle with oregano, salt, and pepper.
4. Bake for 15-20 minutes or until fish is cooked through and vegetables are tender.
5. Serve immediately.

**Tips:**

- Use parchment paper for easy cleanup.
- Add a side of quinoa or brown rice for a more substantial meal.

**Nutritional Values:**
Calories: 210, Fat: 7g, Carbs: 10g, Protein: 30g, Sugar: 3g

## BAKED SALMON WITH ASPARAGUS

**PREP TIME:** 5 min
**COOK TIME:** 15 min
**COOKING METHOD:** Oven
**Servings:** 2

**Ingredients:**

- 2 salmon fillets
- 1 bunch asparagus, trimmed
- 1 tablespoon olive oil
- 1 tablespoon lemon juice
- 1 teaspoon garlic powder

- Salt and pepper to taste

**Steps:**

1. Preheat the oven to 400°F (200°C).
2. Arrange the salmon fillets alongside the asparagus on a baking sheet.
3. Drizzle with olive oil and lemon juice, then add a sprinkle of garlic powder, salt, and pepper for flavor.
4. Bake for 12-15 minutes or until the salmon fully cooked.

**Tips:**
- Serve with a side of brown rice or quinoa for a more substantial meal.

**Nutritional Values:**

Calories: 350, Fat: 20g, Carbs: 6g, Protein: 35g, Sugar: 1g

# SHRIMP STIR-FRY WITH BROCCOLI

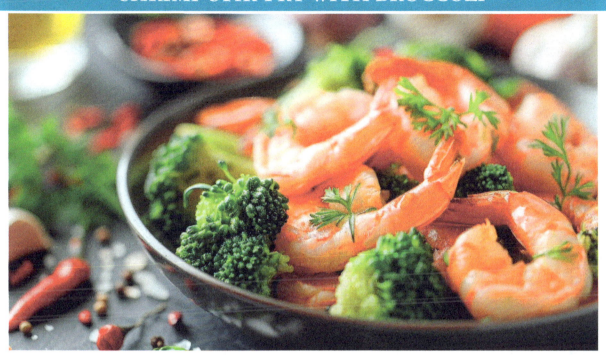

**PREP TIME:** 10 min

**COOK TIME:** 15 min

**COOKING METHOD:** Stovetop

**Servings:** 2

**Ingredients:**
- 1/2 lb shrimp, peeled and deveined
- 1 cup broccoli florets
- 1/2 cup bell peppers, sliced
- 1 tablespoon low-sodium soy sauce
- 1 tablespoon olive oil
- 1 teaspoon ginger, minced
- 1 garlic clove, minced

**Steps:**
1. Heat olive oil in a large pan over medium heat.
2. Add minced garlic and ginger; sauté for 1 minute.
3. Add shrimp and cook until pink, about 3-4 minutes.
4. Add broccoli and bell peppers; stir-fry for another 5-7 minutes.
5. Add soy sauce and cook for 2 more minutes until vegetables are tender.
6. Serve hot.

**Tips:**
- Pair with cauliflower rice for a low-carb meal.
- Add a splash of lemon juice for extra zest.

**Nutritional Values:**

Calories: 156, Fat: 3.3g, Carbs: 6.8g, Protein: 29.4g, Sugar: 1.5g

## BAKED EGGPLANT PARMESAN

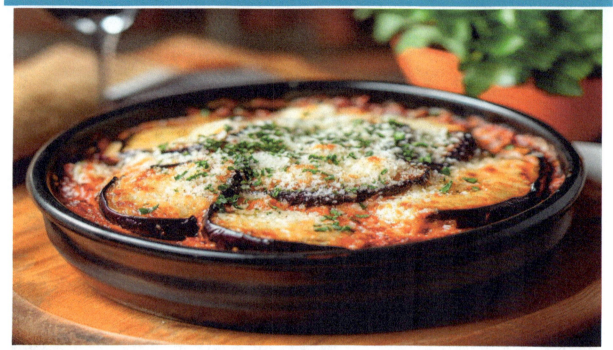

**PREP TIME:** 15 min

**COOK TIME:** 30 min

**COOKING METHOD:** Oven

**Servings:** 4

**Ingredients:**

- 2 medium eggplants, sliced
- 1 cup marinara sauce (low-sodium)
- 1/2 cup low-fat mozzarella cheese, shredded
- 1/4 cup whole wheat breadcrumbs
- 1 tablespoon olive oil
- 1 teaspoon dried basil
- Salt and pepper to taste

**Steps:**

1. Preheat oven to 375°F (190°C).
2. Brush eggplant slices with olive oil and sprinkle with salt and pepper.
3. Arrange in a single layer on a baking sheet and bake for 15 minutes.
4. Layer baked eggplant, marinara sauce, and mozzarella cheese in a baking dish.
5. Sprinkle breadcrumbs on top and bake for another 15 minutes until cheese is melted and bubbly.
6. Serve hot.

**Tips:**

- Serve with a side of whole-grain pasta or salad.
- Use a mandoline slicer for even eggplant slices.

**Nutritional Values:**

Calories: 210, Fat: 9g, Carbs: 25g, Protein: 10g, Sugar: 8g

## QUINOA AND BLACK BEAN BOWL

**PREP TIME:** 5 min

**COOK TIME:** 15 min

**COOKING METHOD:** Stovetop

**Servings:** 2

**Ingredients:**

- 1 cup cooked quinoa
- 1 cup black beans, rinsed and drained
- 1/2 cup sweet corn kernels
- 1/2 avocado, diced
- 1/4 cup fresh cherry tomatoes, halved
- 1 tablespoon of zesty lime juice
- 1 tablespoon olive oil
- 1/2 teaspoon cumin
- Salt and pepper to taste

**Steps:**

1. Put cooked quinoa, black beans, corn, avocado, and cherry tomatoes in a big bowl.
2. Drizzle with lime juice and olive oil.
3. Season with cumin, salt, and pepper, then mix thoroughly.

**Tips:**

- Top with a generous spoonful of Greek yogurt or salsa to enhance the taste.

**Nutritional Values:**

Calories: 300, Fat: 12g, Carbs: 45g, Protein: 12g, Sugar: 6g

## CAULIFLOWER RICE STIR-FRY

**PREP TIME:** 10 min
**COOK TIME:** 10 min
**COOKING METHOD:** Stovetop
Servings: 2
**Ingredients:**

- 2 cups cauliflower rice
- 1/2 cup green peas
- 1/2 cup diced carrots
- 1/2 cup diced bell pepper
- 2 tablespoons low-sodium soy sauce
- 1 tablespoon sesame oil
- 1/2 teaspoon ginger, minced
- 2 cloves garlic, minced
- 1 tablespoon olive oil
- Salt and pepper to taste

**Steps:**

1. Heat olive oil in a skillet over medium heat.
2. Sauté garlic and ginger until fragrant.
3. Incorporate cauliflower rice, peas, carrots, and bell pepper, then stir-fry for 5-7 minutes.
4. Drizzle with sesame oil and soy sauce, then toss to combine.

**Tips:**

- Add a scrambled egg or tofu for additional protein.

**Nutritional Values:**

Calories: 150, Fat: 8g, Carbs: 14g, Protein: 6g, Sugar: 4g

## MEDITERRANEAN CHICKPEA SALAD

**PREP TIME:** 10 min
**COOK TIME:** 0 min
**COOKING METHOD:** No cooking required
Servings: 2
**Ingredients:**

- 1 can chickpeas, rinsed and drained
- 1/2 cucumber, diced
- 1/2 cup cherry tomatoes, halved
- 1/4 red onion, finely chopped
- 1/4 cup Kalamata olives, sliced
- 2 tablespoons of crumbled feta cheese
- 1 tablespoon olive oil
- 1 tablespoon lemon juice
- 1/2 teaspoon oregano
- Salt and pepper to taste

**Steps:**

1. Put chickpeas, cucumber, cherry tomatoes, red onion, and olives in a big bowl.
2. Drizzle with olive oil and lemon juice.
3. Sprinkle with feta cheese, oregano, salt, and pepper, then toss to combine.

**Tips:**

- Serve on a bed of leafy greens for added fiber.

**Nutritional Values:**

Calories: 220, Fat: 10g, Carbs: 28g, Protein: 8g, Sugar: 4g

## GRILLED VEGETABLE WRAP

**PREP TIME:** 10 min
**COOK TIME:** 10 min
**COOKING METHOD:** Grill
**Servings:** 2
**Ingredients:**

- 2 whole wheat tortillas
- 1 zucchini, sliced
- 1 red bell pepper, sliced
- 1/2 eggplant, sliced
- 1 tablespoon olive oil
- 1/4 cup hummus
- Salt and pepper to taste

**Steps:**

1. Brush sliced vegetables with olive oil and season with salt and pepper.
2. Grill vegetables over medium heat until tender.
3. Spread hummus on each tortilla.
4. Layer grilled vegetables on top and roll up the wrap.

**Tips:**

- Add grilled chicken or turkey slices for more protein.

**Nutritional Values:**

Calories: 250, Fat: 10g, Carbs: 30g, Protein: 8g, Sugar: 6g

## SPAGHETTI SQUASH WITH MARINARA SAUCE

**PREP TIME:** 10 min
**COOK TIME:** 40 min
**COOKING METHOD:** Oven
**Servings:** 2
**Ingredients:**

- 1 spaghetti squash, halved and seeded
- 2 cups marinara sauce (no added sugar)
- 1 tablespoon olive oil
- 1/4 cup Parmesan cheese (optional)
- Salt and pepper to taste

**Steps:**

1. Preheat the oven to 400°F (200°C).
2. Brush the cut sides of the squash with olive oil, and season with salt and pepper.
3. Squash halves should be placed cut-side down on a baking pan and baked for 35 to 40 minutes, or until they are soft.
4. Use a fork to scrape the flesh into strands.
5. Warm up the marinara sauce in a skillet and pour it over the spaghetti squash.
6. Sprinkle with Parmesan cheese if desired.

**Tips:**

- Add sautéed vegetables like zucchini or mushrooms to the sauce.

**Nutritional Values:**

Calories: 180, Fat: 7g, Carbs: 28g, Protein: 4g, Sugar: 10g

# QUINOA AND BLACK BEAN SALAD

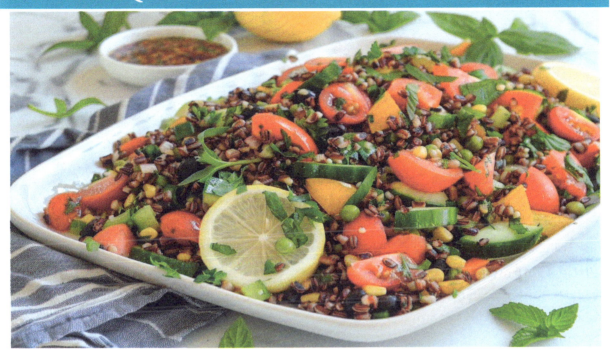

**PREP TIME:** 15 min

**COOK TIME:** 0 min

**COOKING METHOD:** No cooking required

**Servings:** 4

**Ingredients:**

- 1 cup cooked quinoa
- 1 cup black beans, rinsed and drained
- 1/2 cup cherry tomatoes, halved
- 1/2 cup cucumber, diced
- 1/4 cup red onion, diced
- 2 tablespoons olive oil
- 1 tablespoon lime juice
- 1 tablespoon cilantro, chopped
- Salt and pepper to taste

**Steps:**

1. In a large bowl, combine quinoa, black beans, tomatoes, cucumber, and red onion.
2. Drizzle with olive oil, lime juice, cilantro, salt, and pepper.
3. Toss well to combine.
4. Serve chilled or at room temperature.

**Tips:**

- Add avocado for extra creaminess.
- Prepare in advance for a quick meal on busy days.

**Nutritional Values:**

Calories: 200, Fat: 7g, Carbs: 30g, Protein: 8g, Sugar: 2g

# MOROCCAN CHICKPEA STEW

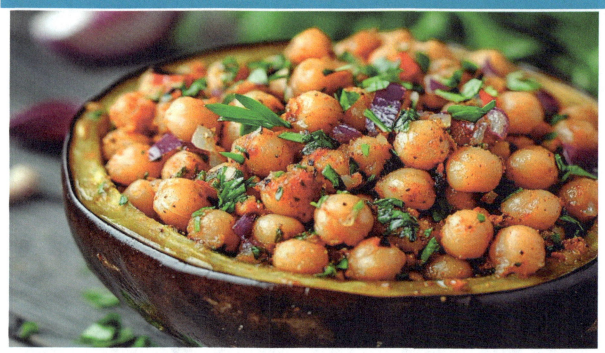

**PREP TIME:** 10 min

**COOK TIME:** 30 min

**COOKING METHOD:** Stovetop

**Servings:** 4

**Ingredients:**

- 1 can chickpeas, rinsed and drained
- 1 large sweet potato, diced
- 1 can diced tomatoes (no salt added)
- 1 onion, diced
- 2 cloves garlic, minced
- 1 teaspoon cumin
- 1/2 teaspoon cinnamon
- 1/4 teaspoon cayenne pepper (optional)
- 1 tablespoon olive oil
- Salt and pepper to taste

**Steps:**

1. Heat olive oil in a pot over medium heat.
2. Sauté onion and garlic until soft.
3. Add sweet potato, tomatoes, chickpeas, cumin, cinnamon, and cayenne.
4. Cover and simmer for 25-30 minutes until sweet potato is tender.
5. Season with salt and pepper.

**Tips:**

- Serve with whole wheat pita or over brown rice.

**Nutritional Values:**

Calories: 220, Fat: 6g, Carbs: 36g, Protein: 6g, Sugar: 10g

# TOFU AND VEGETABLE STIR-FRY

**PREP TIME:** 10 min

**COOK TIME:** 15 min

**COOKING METHOD:** Stovetop

**Servings:** 2

**Ingredients:**

- 1 block firm tofu, cubed
- 1 cup broccoli florets
- 1/2 red bell pepper, sliced
- 1/2 cup snap peas
- 2 tablespoons low-sodium soy sauce
- 1 tablespoon sesame oil
- 1 clove garlic, minced

- 1 tablespoon olive oil
- Salt and pepper to taste

**Steps:**

1. Heat olive oil in a skillet over medium heat.
2. Add tofu cubes and cook until they are golden on all sides.
3. Add garlic, broccoli, bell pepper, and snap peas, and stir-fry for 5-7 minutes.
4. Drizzle with sesame oil and soy sauce, then toss to combine.
5. Season with salt and pepper.

**Tips:**

- Serve over brown rice or quinoa for a complete meal.

**Nutritional Values:**

Calories: 260, Fat: 16g, Carbs: 16g, Protein: 16g, Sugar: 4g

## EGGPLANT AND TOMATO STEW

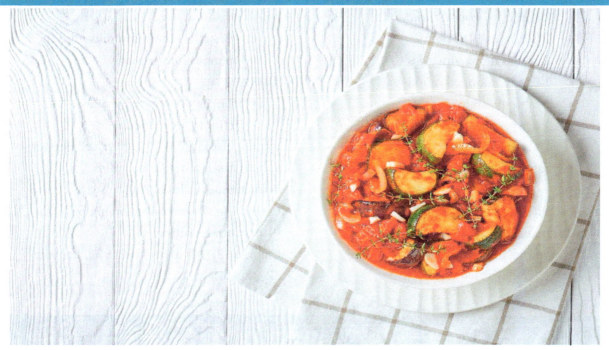

**PREP TIME:** 15 min
**COOK TIME:** 30 min
**COOKING METHOD:** Stovetop
**Servings:** 4
**Ingredients:**

- 1 large eggplant, diced
- 2 tomatoes, diced
- 1 onion, diced
- 3 cloves garlic, minced
- 2 tablespoons olive oil
- 1 teaspoon cumin
- 1/2 teaspoon paprika
- Salt and pepper to taste

**Steps:**

1. Heat olive oil in a pot over medium heat.
2. Sauté onion and garlic until soft.
3. Add eggplant, tomatoes, cumin, and paprika.
4. Cover and let it simmer for 25-30 minutes, stirring occasionally, until the eggplant becomes tender.
5. Season with salt and pepper before serving.

**Tips:**

- Pair it with a delightful serving of whole wheat couscous or quinoa.

**Nutritional Values:**

Calories: 120, Fat: 8g, Carbs: 14g, Protein: 3g, Sugar: 5g

## STUFFED BELL PEPPERS

**PREP TIME:** 15 min
**COOK TIME:** 30 min
**COOKING METHOD:** Oven
**Servings:** 4
**Ingredients:**

- 4 bell peppers, tops cut off and seeds removed
- 1 cup lean ground turkey
- 1/2 cup cooked quinoa
- 1/2 cup diced tomatoes
- 1/2 cup chopped onions
- 1 tablespoon olive oil
- 1 teaspoon cumin
- 1/2 teaspoon paprika
- Salt and pepper to taste

**Steps:**

1. Preheat oven to 375°F (190°C).
2. In a skillet, heat olive oil and sauté onions until soft.
3. Add ground turkey, cumin, paprika, salt, and pepper; cook until the meat is browned.
4. Stir in the diced tomatoes and cooked quinoa.
5. Stuff each bell pepper with the turkey mixture and place in a baking dish.
6. Bake for 25-30 minutes until the peppers are tender.

**Tips:**

- Top with a sprinkle of low-fat cheese for extra flavor.
- Use different colored bell peppers for a more vibrant dish.

**Nutritional Values:** Calories: 180, Fat: 6g, Carbs: 18g, Protein: 18g, Sugar: 6g

**Nutritional Values:**

Calories: 220, Fat: 9g, Carbs: 3g, Protein: 32g, Sugar: 1g

## GRILLED VEGETABLE PLATE

**PREP TIME:** 10 min
**COOK TIME:** 15 min
**COOKING METHOD:** Grill
**Servings:** 2
**Ingredients:**

- 1 zucchini, sliced
- 1 red bell pepper, sliced
- 1 yellow bell pepper, sliced
- 1 red onion, sliced
- 1 tablespoon olive oil
- 1 teaspoon balsamic vinegar
- Salt and pepper to taste

**Steps:**

1. Preheat the grill to medium heat.
2. Toss vegetables with olive oil, balsamic vinegar, salt, and pepper.
3. Grill vegetables for 10-15 minutes, turning occasionally until tender.
4. Serve immediately.

**Tips:**

- Add a sprinkle of feta cheese for extra flavor.
- Serve with grilled chicken or fish for a complete meal.

**Nutritional Values:**

Calories: 100, Fat: 4g, Carbs: 15g, Protein: 2g, Sugar: 6g

1. Sauté onion, carrots, celery, and garlic until softened, about 5-7 minutes.
2. Include minced tomatoes, cumin, paprika, vegetable broth, and lentils.
3. Bring to boil, then lower the heat and let it simmer gently for 25-30 minutes, or until the lentils are soft and tender.
4. Season with salt and pepper prior to serving.

**Tips:**
- Pair with a side salad or whole-grain crackers for a balanced meal.

**Nutritional Values:**

Calories: 180, Fat: 4g, Carbs: 32g, Protein: 10g, Sugar: 7g

## ZUCCHINI NOODLES WITH MARINARA SAUCE

**PREP TIME:** 10 min
**COOK TIME:** 10 min
**COOKING METHOD:** Stovetop
**Servings:** 2
**Ingredients:**
- 2 medium zucchinis, spiralized into noodles
- 1 cup marinara sauce (low-sodium)
- 1 tablespoon olive oil
- 1/2 teaspoon Italian seasoning
- 1/4 teaspoon red pepper flakes (optional)
- Salt and pepper to taste

**Steps:**
1. Heat olive oil in a pan over medium heat.
2. Add zucchini noodles and sauté for 2-3 minutes until slightly tender.
3. Add marinara sauce, Italian seasoning, red pepper flakes, salt, and pepper.
4. Cook for another 5 minutes until the sauce is heated.
5. Serve immediately.

**Tips:**
- Add grilled chicken or shrimp for extra protein.
- Use a vegetable spiralizer to make fresh zucchini noodles easily.

**Nutritional Values:**

Calories: 120, Fat: 7g, Carbs: 12g, Protein: 3g, Sugar: 5g

# LENTIL AND VEGETABLE SOUP

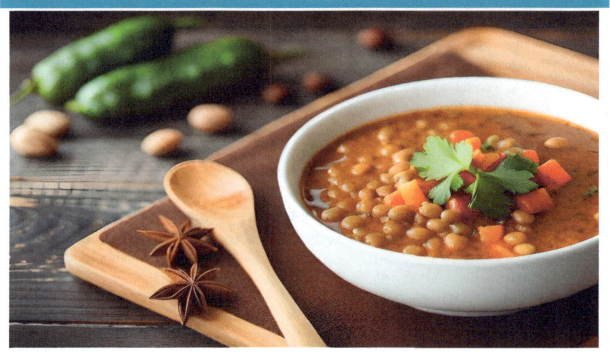

**PREP TIME:** 15 min

**COOK TIME:** 30 min

**COOKING METHOD:** Stovetop

Servings: 4

Ingredients:

- 1 cup dry lentils, rinsed
- 1 medium onion, diced
- 2 carrots, diced
- 2 celery stalks, diced
- 3 cloves garlic, minced
- 1 can diced tomatoes (no salt added)
- 4 cups low-sodium vegetable broth
- 1 teaspoon cumin
- 1/2 teaspoon paprika
- 1 tablespoon olive oil
- Salt and pepper to taste

Steps:

5. In a large pot, heat olive oil over medium heat.

6. Sauté onion, carrots, celery, and garlic until softened, about 5-7 minutes.

7. Include minced tomatoes, cumin, paprika, vegetable broth, and lentils.

8. Bring to boil, then lower the heat and let it simmer gently for 25-30 minutes, or until the lentils are soft and tender.

9. Season with salt and pepper prior to serving.

**Tips:**

- Pair with a side salad or whole-grain crackers for a balanced meal.

**Nutritional Values:**

Calories: 180, Fat: 4g, Carbs: 32g, Protein: 10g, Sugar: 7g

# CHAPTER 8: HEALTHY SNACKS

## GREEK YOGURT AND BERRY BOWL

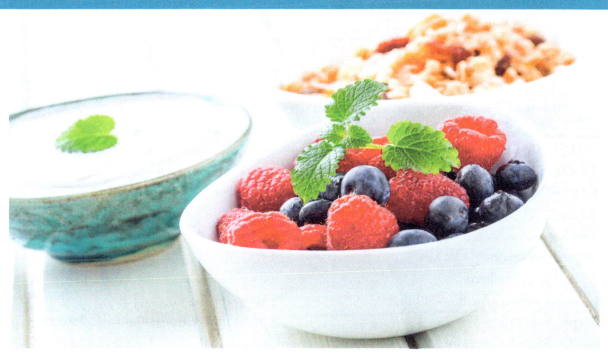

**PREP TIME:** 5 min

**COOK TIME:** 0 min

**COOKING METHOD:** No cooking required

**Servings:** 1

**Ingredients:**

- 1/2 cup plain Greek yogurt
- 1/2 cup mixed berries (strawberries, blueberries, raspberries)
- 1 teaspoon honey

**Steps:**

1. In a bowl, combine Greek yogurt and mixed berries.
2. Drizzle honey over the top and mix gently.
3. Serve immediately.

**Tips:**

- Add a tablespoon of chia seeds for extra fiber.
- Use frozen berries for a cooler snack.

**Nutritional Values:**

Calories: 120, Fat: 2g, Carbs: 15g, Protein: 10g, Sugar: 10g

## CUCUMBER HUMMUS BITES

**PREP TIME:** 10 min

**COOK TIME:** 0 min

**COOKING METHOD:** No cooking required

**Servings:** 2

**Ingredients:**

- 1 cucumber, sliced into rounds
- 1/2 cup hummus
- 1 tablespoon chopped parsley

**Steps:**

1. Arrange cucumber slices on a plate.
2. Top each cucumber slice with a dollop of hummus.
3. Sprinkle with chopped parsley and serve immediately.

**Tips:**

- Add a sprinkle of paprika or red pepper flakes for a spicy kick.
- Use different flavored hummus to add variety.

**Nutritional Values:**

Calories: 70, Fat: 3g, Carbs: 8g, Protein: 2g, Sugar: 2g

## APPLE SLICES WITH ALMOND BUTTER

**PREP TIME:** 5 min
**COOK TIME:** 0 min
**COOKING METHOD:** No cooking required
**Servings:** 1
**Ingredients:**

- 1 apple, sliced
- 1 tablespoon almond butter

**Steps:**

1. Slice the apple into thin rounds.
2. Spread almond butter evenly on each apple slice.
3. Serve immediately.

**Tips:**

- Sprinkle cinnamon on top for extra flavor.
- Use pear slices as an alternative to apples.

**Nutritional Values:** Calories: 150, Fat: 7g, Carbs: 20g, Protein: 3g, Sugar: 15g

## CARROT STICKS WITH GREEK YOGURT DIP

**PREP TIME:** 5 min
**COOK TIME:** 0 min
**COOKING METHOD:** No cooking required
**Servings:** 2
**Ingredients:**

- 1 cup carrot sticks
- 1/2 cup plain Greek yogurt
- 1 tablespoon lemon juice
- 1/2 teaspoon dill

**Steps:**

1. In a small bowl, mix Greek yogurt, lemon juice, and dill.
2. Serve the yogurt dip with carrot sticks.

**Tips:**

- Substitute cucumber or celery sticks for variety.
- Add a pinch of garlic powder to the dip for extra flavor.

**Nutritional Values:**

Calories: 90, Fat: 1g, Carbs: 12g, Protein: 7g, Sugar: 6g

# HARD-BOILED EGGS WITH PAPRIKA

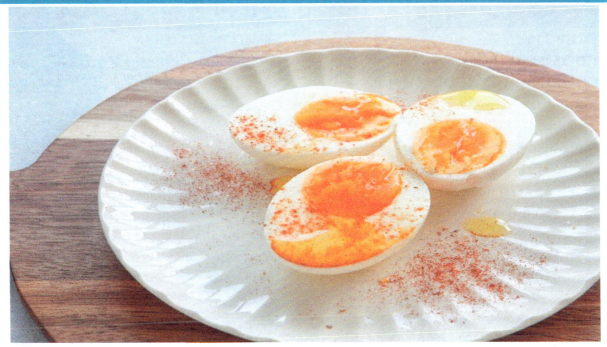

**PREP TIME:** 5 min

**COOK TIME:** 10 min

**COOKING METHOD:** Stovetop

**Servings:** 2

**Ingredients:**

- 2 large eggs
- 1/4 teaspoon paprika
- Salt and pepper to taste

**Steps:**

1. Boil the eggs in a pot of water for 10 minutes.
2. Cool, peel, and slice the eggs in half.
3. Sprinkle with paprika, salt, and pepper.

**Tips:**

- Prepare a batch of hard-boiled eggs in advance for easy snacking.
- Add a dash of hot sauce for a spicy kick.

**Nutritional Values:**

Calories: 140, Fat: 9g, Carbs: 1g, Protein: 12g, Sugar: 0g

# CELERY STICKS WITH LOW-FAT CREAM CHEESE

**PREP TIME:** 5 min

**COOK TIME:** 0 min

**COOKING METHOD:** No cooking required

**Servings:** 2

**Ingredients:**

- 4 celery sticks
- 2 tablespoons low-fat cream cheese

**Steps:**

1. Spread cream cheese inside each celery stick.
2. Serve immediately.

**Tips:**

- Top with chopped chives or nuts for extra crunch.
- Substitute with low-fat cottage cheese for a different texture.

**Nutritional Values:** Calories: 70, Fat: 4g, Carbs: 4g, Protein: 2g, Sugar: 1g

## COTTAGE CHEESE WITH PINEAPPLE

**PREP TIME:** 5 min

**COOK TIME:** 0 min

**COOKING METHOD:** No cooking required

**Servings:** 1

**Ingredients:**

- 1/2 cup low-fat cottage cheese
- 1/4 cup pineapple chunks (fresh or canned in water)

**Steps:**

1. Combine cottage cheese and pineapple in a bowl.
2. Serve immediately.

**Tips:**

- Use other fruits like peaches or berries for variety.
- Add a sprinkle of cinnamon for added flavor.

**Nutritional Values:**

Calories: 100, Fat: 2g, Carbs: 14g, Protein: 10g, Sugar: 9g

## MINI BELL PEPPERS WITH HUMMUS

**PREP TIME:** 5 min

**COOK TIME:** 0 min

**COOKING METHOD:** No cooking required

**Servings:** 2

**Ingredients:**

- 6 mini bell peppers, halved and seeded
- 1/2 cup hummus

**Steps:**

1. Spoon hummus into each bell pepper half.
2. Arrange on a plate and serve.

**Tips:**

- Garnish with chopped parsley or cilantro for extra freshness.
- Use different hummus flavors to mix things up.

**Nutritional Values:**

Calories: 90, Fat: 3g, Carbs: 12g, Protein: 3g, Sugar: 3g

# ZUCCHINI CHIPS

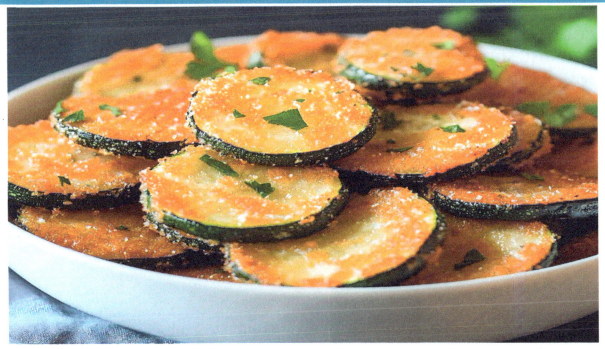

**PREP TIME:** 10 min

**COOK TIME:** 40 min

**COOKING METHOD:** Oven

**Servings:** 2

**Ingredients:**

- 1 zucchini, thinly sliced
- 1 tablespoon olive oil
- Salt and pepper to taste

**Steps:**

1. Preheat the oven to 225°F (110°C).
2. Toss zucchini slices with olive oil, salt, and pepper.
3. Arrange on a baking sheet in a single layer.
4. Bake for 40 minutes or until crisp.

**Tips:**

- Use a mandoline for even slices.
- Sprinkle with Parmesan for extra flavor.

**Nutritional Values:**

Calories: 70, Fat: 4g, Carbs: 7g, Protein: 2g, Sugar: 3g

# EDAMAME WITH SEA SALT

**PREP TIME:** 5 min

**COOK TIME:** 5 min

**COOKING METHOD:** Stovetop

**Servings:** 2

**Ingredients:**

- 1 cup shelled edamame
- 1/2 teaspoon sea salt

**Steps:**

1. Boil edamame in salted water for 5 minutes.
2. Drain and sprinkle with sea salt.
3. Serve immediately.

**Tips:**

- Toss with a little olive oil and chili flakes for a spicy version.
- Serve hot or cold as per preference.

**Nutritional Values:** Calories: 120, Fat: 5g, Carbs: 10g, Protein: 12g, Sugar: 2g

## OVEN-ROASTED CHICKPEAS

**PREP TIME:** 5 min
**COOK TIME:** 40 min
**COOKING METHOD:** Oven
**Servings:** 2
**Ingredients:**

- 1 cup chickpeas, rinsed and drained
- 1 tablespoon olive oil
- 1 teaspoon paprika
- Salt to taste

**Steps:**

1. Preheat the oven to 400°F (200°C).
2. Toss chickpeas with olive oil, paprika, and salt.
3. Spread on a baking sheet in a single layer.
4. Bake for 40 minutes or until crispy.

**Tips:**

- Add garlic powder or cumin for extra flavor.
- Store in an airtight container for up to a week.

**Nutritional Values:**

Calories: 130, Fat: 4g, Carbs: 20g, Protein: 5g, Sugar: 1g

## BAKED KALE CHIPS

**PREP TIME:** 5 min
**COOK TIME:** 15 min
**COOKING METHOD:** Oven
**Servings:** 2
**Ingredients:**

- 2 cups kale leaves, torn into pieces
- 1 tablespoon olive oil
- Salt to taste

**Steps:**

1. Preheat the oven to 350°F (175°C).
2. Toss kale leaves with olive oil and salt.
3. Spread on a baking sheet in a single layer.
4. Bake for 10-15 minutes until crispy.

**Tips:**

- Add a pinch of cayenne pepper for a spicy kick.
- Use nutritional yeast for a cheesy flavor without added fat.

**Nutritional Values:**

Calories: 50, Fat: 3g, Carbs: 6g, Protein: 2g, Sugar: 1g

## TURKEY ROLL-UPS

**PREP TIME:** 5 min
**COOK TIME:** 0 min
**COOKING METHOD:** No cooking required
**Servings:** 2
**Ingredients:**

- 4 slices turkey breast
- 2 slices low-fat cheese
- 4 spinach leaves

**Steps:**

1. Place cheese and spinach leaves on each turkey slice.
2. Roll up tightly and serve.

**Tips:**

- Secure with toothpicks for easy handling.
- Add mustard or hummus for extra flavor.

**Nutritional Values:**

Calories: 110, Fat: 3g, Carbs: 2g, Protein: 15g, Sugar: 1g

# COTTAGE CHEESE AND CUCUMBER SLICES

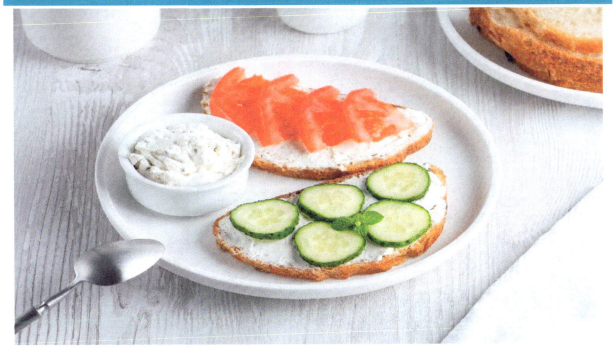

**PREP TIME:** 5 min

**COOK TIME:** 0 min

**COOKING METHOD:** No cooking required

**Servings:** 1

**Ingredients:**

- 1/2 cup low-fat cottage cheese
- 1/2 cucumber, sliced

**Steps:**

1. Serve cottage cheese with cucumber slices on the side.

2. Sprinkle with black pepper or herbs for added flavor.

**Tips:**

- Add a drizzle of balsamic vinegar for a tangy twist.
- Substitute with tomatoes or radishes for variety.

**Nutritional Values:** Calories: 80, Fat: 1g, Carbs: 6g, Protein: 12g, Sugar: 4g

# ALMOND AND RAISIN MIX

**PREP TIME:** 2 min

**COOK TIME:** 0 min

**COOKING METHOD:** No cooking required

**Servings:** 2

**Ingredients:**

- 1/4 cup almonds
- 1/4 cup raisins

**Steps:**

1. Mix almonds and raisins in a bowl.

2. Serve immediately or pack in a small container for on-the-go.

**Tips:**

- Add other nuts or dried fruits for variety.
- Portion control is key; limit servings to avoid excess calories.

**Nutritional Values:**

Calories: 150, Fat: 7g, Carbs: 20g, Protein: 3g, Sugar: 12g

# TOMATO BASIL BITES

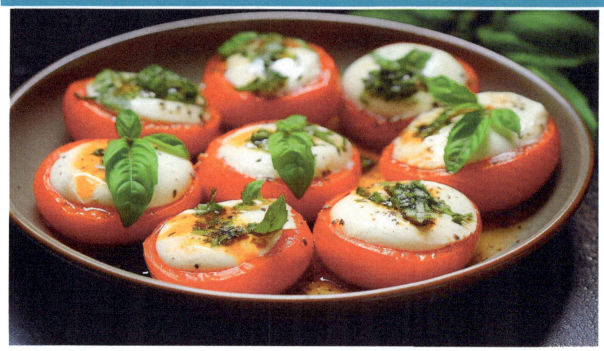

**PREP TIME:** 5 min

**COOK TIME:** 0 min

**COOKING METHOD:** No cooking required

**Servings:** 2

**Ingredients:**

- 1 large tomato, sliced
- 1/4 cup fresh basil leaves
- 1/4 cup low-fat mozzarella, sliced

**Steps:**

1. Arrange tomato slices on a plate.
2. Top each slice with basil leaves and mozzarella.
3. Serve immediately.

**Tips:**

- Drizzle with balsamic glaze for extra flavor.
- Use cherry tomatoes for a bite-sized version.

**Nutritional Values:**

Calories: 80, Fat: 3g, Carbs: 6g, Protein: 5g, Sugar: 3g

# MIXED BERRY POPSICLES

**PREP TIME:** 10 min (plus freezing time)

**COOK TIME:** 0 min

**COOKING METHOD:** No cooking required

**Servings:** 4

**Ingredients:**

- 1 cup mixed berries
- 1/2 cup plain Greek yogurt
- 1 tablespoon honey

**Steps:**

1. Blend berries, yogurt, and honey until smooth.
2. Pour into popsicle molds and freeze for 4 hours or until solid.

**Tips:**

- Use silicone molds for easy removal.
- Add a few whole berries to each mold for extra texture.

**Nutritional Values:**

Calories: 70, Fat: 1g, Carbs: 13g, Protein: 3g,
Sugar: 10g

## SPICED NUTS

**PREP TIME:** 5 min

**COOK TIME:** 10 min

**COOKING METHOD:** Stovetop

**Servings:** 2

**Ingredients:**

- 1/2 cup mixed nuts (almonds, walnuts, cashews)
- 1/2 teaspoon paprika
- 1/2 teaspoon cumin
- 1/2 teaspoon garlic powder
- 1 teaspoon olive oil

**Steps:**

1. Heat olive oil in a skillet over medium heat.
2. Add nuts and spices; stir continuously for 5-7 minutes until fragrant.
3. Allow to cool before serving.

**Tips:**

- Store in an airtight container for a week.
- Mix with seeds or dried fruit for added variety.

**Nutritional Values:** Calories:
180, Fat: 15g, Carbs: 8g, Protein: 5g, Sugar: 2g

# CHAPTER 9: SMOOTHIES & HYDRATION DRINKS

## ICED HERBAL TEA

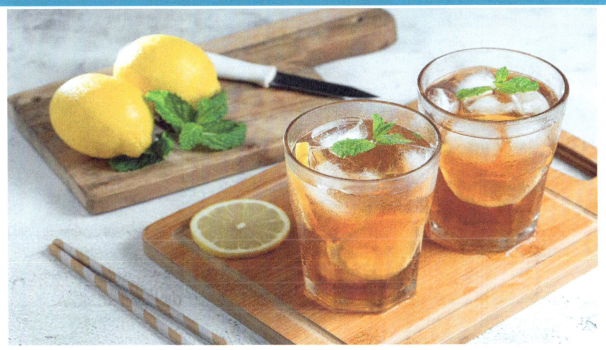

**PREP TIME:** 5 min (plus steeping time)

**COOK TIME:** 0 min

**COOKING METHOD:** Stovetop

**Servings:** 4

**Ingredients:**

- 4 cups water
- 4 herbal tea bags (e.g., chamomile, peppermint)
- Lemon slices (optional)
- Ice cubes

**Steps:**

1. Boil water and steep tea bags for 5-7 minutes.
2. Let cool, then pour over ice in glasses.
3. Garnish with lemon slices if desired.

**Tips:**

- Experiment with different herbal teas for varied flavors.
- Sweeten with a touch of honey if needed.

**Nutritional Values:**

Calories: 5, Fat: 0g, Carbs: 1g, Protein: 0g, Sugar: 0g

## BERRY SMOOTHIE

**PREP TIME:** 5 min

**COOK TIME:** 0 min

**COOKING METHOD:** No cooking required

**Servings:** 1

**Ingredients:**

- 1 cup mixed berries (strawberries, blueberries, raspberries)
- 1/2 cup **unsweetened** and unflavored almond milk
- 1/2 cup plain **non-fat** Greek yogurt

- 1/4 teaspoon vanilla extract

**Steps:**

1. In a blender, combine the mixed berries, almond milk, Greek yogurt, and vanilla extract.
2. Mix until it's creamy and smooth.
3. Pour it into a glass and serve right away.

**Tips:**

Add a handful of spinach or kale for added nutrition. Use frozen berries for a thicker smoothie.

**Nutritional Values:**

Calories: 130, Fat: 3g, Carbs: 15g, Protein: 10g, Sugar: 8g

## CUCUMBER LIME REFRESHER

**PREP TIME:** 5 min
**COOK TIME:** 0 min
**COOKING METHOD:** No cooking required
**Servings:** 2
**Ingredients:**

- 1 cucumber, sliced
- 1 lime, sliced
- 1-liter sparkling water
- Ice cubes (optional)

**Steps:**

1. Add cucumber and lime slices to a pitcher.
2. Pour sparkling water over the ingredients and stir gently.
3. Serve immediately over ice.

**Tips:**

- Add a splash of unsweetened coconut water for a tropical twist.
- Use a flavored sparkling water (no added sugar) for extra taste.

**Nutritional Values:**

Calories: 5, Fat: 0g, Carbs: 2g, Protein: 0g, Sugar: 0g

## BERRY GREEN SMOOTHIE

**PREP TIME:** 5 min
**COOK TIME:** 10 min
**COOKING METHOD:** Blender required
**Servings:** 1
**Ingredients:**

- 1/2 cup spinach
- 1/2 cup mixed berries (strawberries, blueberries, raspberries)
- 1/2 cup unsweetened almond milk
- 1 tablespoon chia seeds
- 1/2 teaspoon honey (optional)

**Steps:**

1. Combine all ingredients in a blender and blend until smooth.
2. Pour into a glass and serve immediately.

**Tips:**

- Add a few ice cubes to make the smoothie colder and thicker.
- Use kale instead of spinach for a different green option.

**Nutritional Values:**

Calories: 90, Fat: 3g, Carbs: 15g, Protein: 2g, Sugar: 6g

## APPLE CIDER VINEGAR TONIC

**PREP TIME:** 5 min
**COOK TIME:** 10 min
**COOKING METHOD:** No cooking required
**Servings:** 1
**Ingredients:**

- 1 tablespoon apple cider vinegar
- 1 cup water
- 1/2 teaspoon honey (optional)
- Ice cubes (optional)

**Steps:**

1. Mix apple cider vinegar, water, and honey in a glass.
2. Stir well and serve over ice if desired.

**Tips:**

- Start with a small amount of vinegar to get used to the taste.
- Add a splash of lemon juice for extra flavor.

**Nutritional Values:**
Calories: 10, Fat: 0g, Carbs: 3g, Protein: 0g, Sugar: 2g

## MATCHA GREEN TEA LATTE

**PREP TIME:** 5 min
**COOK TIME:** 10 min
**COOKING METHOD:** No cooking required
**Servings:** 1
**Ingredients:**

- 1 teaspoon matcha green tea powder
- 1/2 cup hot water
- 1/2 cup unsweetened almond milk, warmed
- 1/2 teaspoon honey (optional)

**Steps:**

1. Whisk matcha powder with hot water until frothy.
2. Stir in warmed almond milk and honey, if using.
3. Serve immediately.

**Tips:**

- Use a matcha whisk for a smoother consistency.
- Substitute almond milk with coconut milk for a different flavor.

**Nutritional Values:**
Calories: 30, Fat: 1g, Carbs: 5g, Protein: 1g, Sugar: 3g

## COCONUT WATER ELECTROLYTE DRINK

**PREP TIME:** 5 min
**COOK TIME:** 10 min
**COOKING METHOD:** No cooking required
**Servings:** 2
**Ingredients:**

- 2 cups unsweetened coconut water
- 1/2 cup orange juice (freshly squeezed)
- Pinch of sea salt

**Steps:**

1. Mix coconut water, orange juice, and sea salt in a pitcher.
2. Serve over ice.

**Tips:**

- Add a slice of lemon or lime for extra zest.

- Perfect after a workout to replenish electrolytes.

**Nutritional Values:**
Calories: 50, Fat: 0g, Carbs: 12g, Protein: 1g, Sugar: 10g

## WATERMELON COOLER

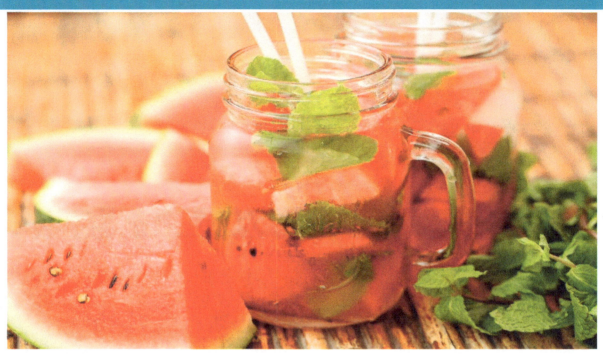

**PREP TIME:** 5 min

**COOKING METHOD:** Blender required

**Servings:** 2

**Ingredients:**
- 2 cups watermelon, cubed
- Juice of 1 lime
- Fresh mint leaves
- Ice cubes

**Steps:**
1. Blend watermelon and lime juice until smooth.
2. Serve over ice with fresh mint leaves.

**Tips:**
- For added texture, include a few whole watermelon cubes in the drink.
- Use a combination of watermelon and cucumber for extra hydration.

**Nutritional Values:**
Calories: 30, Fat: 0g, Carbs: 8g, Protein: 1g, Sugar: 6g

## CINNAMON ALMOND MILK

**PREP TIME:** 5 min

**COOK TIME:** 10 min

**COOKING METHOD:** Stovetop

**Servings:** 2

**Ingredients:**
- 2 cups unsweetened almond milk
- 1/2 teaspoon ground cinnamon
- 1/2 teaspoon vanilla extract
- 1 teaspoon honey (optional)

**Steps:**
1. Heat almond milk in a small saucepan until warm.
2. Stir in cinnamon, vanilla extract, and honey.

3. Serve warm or chilled.

**Tips:**

- Use a frother to create a latte-like texture.

- Add a dash of nutmeg or ginger for a spiced version.

**Nutritional Values:**

Calories: 40, Fat: 2g, Carbs: 5g, Protein: 1g, Sugar: 3g

## 9.1 DETOX ELIXIRS

### TURMERIC GINGER TEA

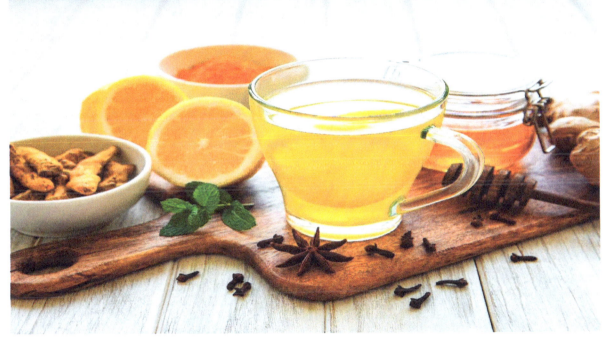

**PREP TIME:** 5 min

**COOK TIME:** 10 min

**COOKING METHOD:** Stovetop

**Servings: 2**

**Ingredients:**

- 2 cups water
- 1/2 teaspoon ground turmeric
- 1/2 teaspoon grated ginger
- 1 teaspoon lemon juice
- 1/2 teaspoon honey (optional)

**Steps:**

1. Bring water to a boil in a small saucepan.

2. Add turmeric and ginger, then simmer for 5 minutes.

3. Strain the tea, add lemon juice and honey, and serve warm.

**Tips:**

- Add a pinch of black pepper to enhance turmeric absorption.

- Enjoy chilled over ice for a refreshing version.

**Nutritional Values:**

Calories: 10, Fat: 0g, Carbs: 2g, Protein: 0g, Sugar: 1g

## LEMON MINT DETOX WATER

**PREP TIME:** 5 min

**COOK TIME:** 0 min

**COOKING METHOD:** No cooking required

**Servings:** 4

**Ingredients:**

- 1 lemon, thinly sliced
- 10 fresh mint leaves
- 1-liter water
- Ice cubes (optional)

**Steps:**

1. In a large pitcher, add lemon slices and mint leaves.
2. Pour water over the ingredients and let it infuse for at least 30 minutes.
3. Serve chilled with ice cubes if desired.

**Tips:**

- For added flavor, include cucumber slices or a few berries.
- Prepare in advance and store in the refrigerator for a refreshing drink throughout the day.

**Nutritional Values:**

Calories: 5, Fat: 0g, Carbs: 1g, Protein: 0g, Sugar: 0g

## GREEN TEA WITH LEMON

**PREP TIME:** 5 min

**COOK TIME:** 0 min

**COOKING METHOD:** Stovetop

**Servings:** 4

**Ingredients:**

- 4 cups water
- 4 green tea bags or 4 teaspoons loose green tea
- 1 lemon, sliced

**Steps:**

1. Boil water and steep green tea for 3-5 minutes.
2. Add lemon slices for extra flavor and vitamin C.
3. Serve warm or over ice.

**Tips:**

- Sweeten with honey if desired.
- Great for digestion after meals.

**Nutritional Values:**

Calories: 5, Fat: 0g, Carbs: 1g, Protein: 0g, Sugar: 0g

## LEMON GINGER WATER

**PREP TIME:** 5 min (plus steeping time)

**COOK TIME:** 0 min

**COOKING METHOD:** No cooking required

**Servings:** 4

**Ingredients:**

- 1 lemon, juiced
- 1-inch piece of ginger, grated
- 4 cups water

**Steps:**

1. Add the lemon juice and grated ginger to a pitcher of water.
2. Let it steep for at least 30 minutes before drinking.
3. Serve chilled or at room temperature.

**Tips:**

- Drink first thing in the morning to kick-start digestion.

- Add a touch of honey for sweetness if needed.

**Nutritional Values:**
Calories: 5, Fat: 0g, Carbs: 1g, Protein: 0g, Sugar: 0g

# CUCUMBER LIME DETOX WATER

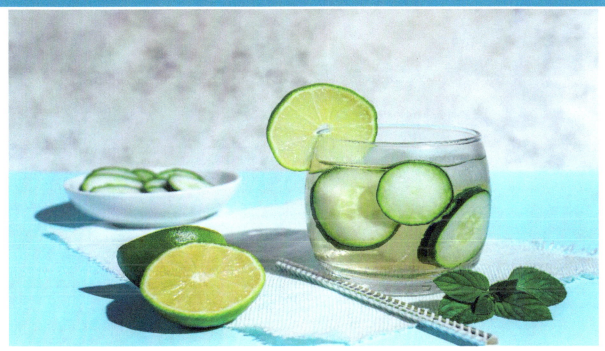

**PREP TIME:** 5 min (plus steeping time)
**COOK TIME:** 0 min
**COOKING METHOD:** No cooking required
**Servings:** 4
**Ingredients:**
- 1 cucumber, thinly sliced
- 1 lime, thinly sliced
- 4 cups water

**Steps:**
1. Add cucumber and lime slices to a pitcher of water.
2. Let it steep in the fridge for a few hours.
3. Serve chilled.

**Tips:**
- Add a few fresh mint leaves for extra flavor.
- Sip throughout the day to stay hydrated.

**Nutritional Values:**
Calories: 5, Fat: 0g, Carbs: 1g, Protein: 0g, Sugar: 0g

# CHAPTER 10: DESSERTS

## BAKED APPLES WITH CINNAMON

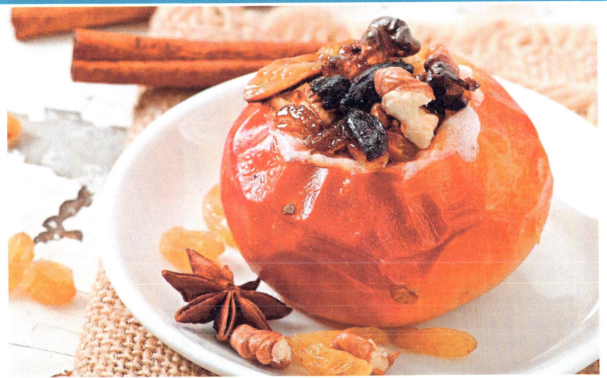

**PREP TIME:** 10 min
**COOK TIME:** 20 min
**COOKING METHOD:** Oven
**Servings:** 2
**Ingredients:**

- 2 medium apples, cored
- 1/2 teaspoon ground cinnamon
- 1/4 teaspoon nutmeg
- 1 tablespoon raisins
- 1 teaspoon honey

**Steps:**

1. Preheat the oven to 350°F (175°C).
2. Place cored apples on a baking sheet.
3. Sprinkle cinnamon and nutmeg inside each apple.
4. Stuff each apple with raisins and drizzle with honey.
5. Bake for 20 minutes or until tender.

**Tips:**

- Serve with a dollop of Greek yogurt for extra creaminess.
- Use a mix of different apples for varied flavors.

**Nutritional Values:**

Calories: 110, Fat: 0g, Carbs: 28g, Protein: 1g, Sugar: 22g

## BANANA NICE CREAM

**PREP TIME:** 5 min (plus freezing time)
**COOK TIME:** 0 min
**COOKING METHOD:** No cooking required
**Servings:** 2
**Ingredients:**

- 2 ripe bananas, sliced and frozen
- 1/2 teaspoon vanilla extract

**Steps:**

1. Blend frozen banana slices and vanilla extract in a food processor until smooth and creamy.

2. Serve immediately as a soft-serve or freeze for an additional hour for a firmer texture.

Tips:

- Add a tablespoon of cocoa powder for a chocolate version.

- Mix in a handful of berries or nuts for extra texture.

**Nutritional Values:**

Calories: 100, Fat: 0g, Carbs: 27g, Protein: 1g, Sugar: 14g

## POACHED PEARS WITH CINNAMON

**PREP TIME:** 10 min
**COOK TIME:** 15 min
**COOKING METHOD:** Stovetop
Servings: 2
Ingredients:

- 2 pears, peeled and halved
- 1 cup water
- 1/2 teaspoon ground cinnamon
- 1 teaspoon honey

Steps:

1. In a saucepan, bring water, cinnamon, and honey to a boil.
2. Add pears and reduce heat to a simmer.

3. Cook for 15 minutes or until pears are tender.
4. Serve warm with a drizzle of the poaching liquid.

Tips:

- Use a cinnamon stick instead of ground cinnamon for a more intense flavor.
- Add a dash of nutmeg or cloves for added spice.

**Nutritional Values:**

Calories: 90, Fat: 0g, Carbs: 24g, Protein: 1g, Sugar: 18g

## OAT AND BERRY CRISP

**PREP TIME:** 10 min
**COOK TIME:** 20 min
**COOKING METHOD:** Oven
Servings: 4
Ingredients:

- 2 cups mixed berries
- 1/2 cup rolled oats
- 2 tablespoons almond flour
- 1 tablespoon honey
- 1/2 teaspoon cinnamon

Steps:

1. Preheat the oven to 350°F (175°C).
2. In a bowl, mix oats, almond flour, honey, and cinnamon.

3. Spread berries in a baking dish and sprinkle the oat mixture on top.
4. Bake for 20 minutes or until the top is golden and crispy.

Tips:

- Use different types of fruit, like apples or peaches, for variety.
- Serve with a dollop of Greek yogurt or a scoop of banana nice cream.

**Nutritional Values:**

Calories: 120, Fat: 3g, Carbs: 22g, Protein: 3g, Sugar: 10g

# CHOCOLATE AVOCADO MOUSSE

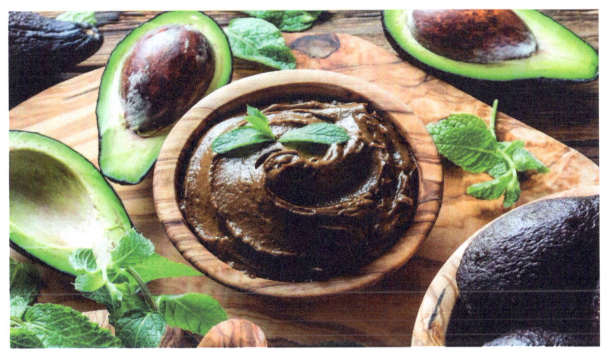

**PREP TIME:** 10 min

**COOK TIME:** 0 min

**COOKING METHOD:** No cooking required

**Servings:** 2

**Ingredients:**

- 1 ripe avocado
- 2 tablespoons unsweetened cocoa powder
- 2 tablespoons honey
- 1/2 teaspoon vanilla extract

**Steps:**

1. In a blender, combine avocado, cocoa powder, honey, and vanilla extract.
2. Blend until smooth and creamy.
3. Chill in the refrigerator for 30 minutes before serving.

**Tips:**

- Garnish with fresh berries or a dollop of Greek yogurt.
- Adjust sweetness to taste by adding more or less honey.

**Nutritional Values:**

Calories: 160, Fat: 10g, Carbs: 20g, Protein: 2g, Sugar: 15g

# STRAWBERRY SORBET

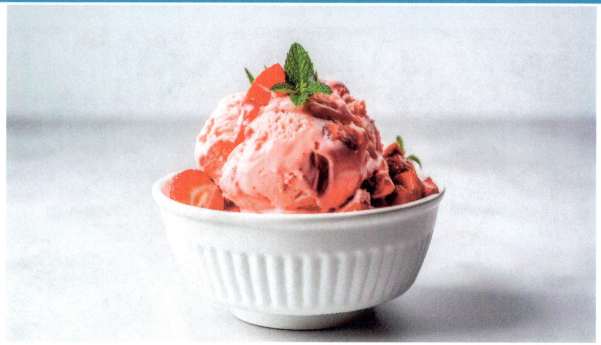

**PREP TIME:** 5 min (plus freezing time)

**COOK TIME:** 0 min

**COOKING METHOD**: No cooking required

**Servings:** 4

**Ingredients:**

- 2 cups strawberries, hulled and frozen
- 1 tablespoon lemon juice
- 1 tablespoon honey

**Steps:**

1. Blend strawberries, lemon juice, and honey in a food processor until smooth.
2. Freeze for at least 2 hours before serving.

**Tips:**

- Add a few fresh mint leaves for a refreshing twist.
- Use any other type of berry or fruit to change the flavor.

**Nutritional Values:**

Calories: 60, Fat: 0g, Carbs: 16g, Protein: 1g, Sugar: 10g

# CINNAMON APPLE CHIPS

**PREP TIME:** 10 min
**COOK TIME:** 1 hour
**COOKING METHOD:** Oven
**Servings:** 2
**Ingredients:**

- 2 apples, thinly sliced
- 1/2 teaspoon ground cinnamon

**Steps:**

1. Preheat oven to 225°F (110°C).
2. Arrange apple slices on a baking sheet lined with parchment paper.
3. Sprinkle with cinnamon.
4. Bake for 1 hour or until the chips are crisp.

**Tips:**

- Use a mandoline slicer for even, thin slices.
- Store in an airtight container to keep them crisp.

**Nutritional Values:**

Calories: 60, Fat: 0g, Carbs: 16g, Protein: 0g, Sugar: 12g

# BERRY COMPOTE WITH YOGURT

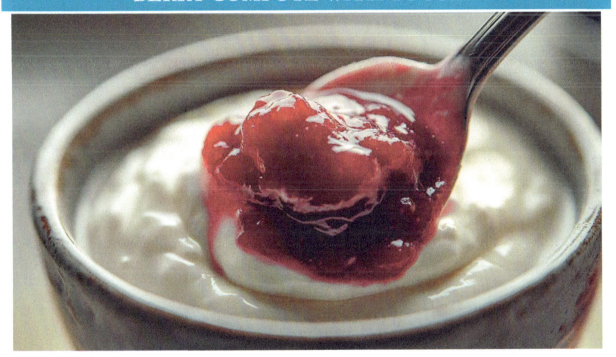

**PREP TIME:** 5 min
**COOK TIME:** 10 min
**COOKING METHOD:** Stovetop
**Servings:** 2
**Ingredients:**

- 1 cup mixed berries (strawberries, blueberries, raspberries)
- 1 tablespoon water
- 1 teaspoon honey
- 1/2 cup plain Greek yogurt

**Steps:**

1. In a small saucepan, combine berries, water, and honey.
2. Simmer over medium heat until the berries break down and form a sauce (about 10 minutes).
3. Serve the compote over Greek yogurt.

**Tips:**

- Add a pinch of cinnamon or vanilla extract for added flavor.

- Use frozen berries if fresh are not available.

## COCONUT MILK PANNA COTTA

**PREP TIME:** 10 min (plus chilling time)
**COOK TIME:** 5 min
**COOKING METHOD:** Stovetop
**Servings:** 2
**Ingredients:**

- 1 cup unsweetened coconut milk
- 1 tablespoon gelatin
- 2 tablespoons honey
- 1/2 teaspoon vanilla extract

**Steps:**

1. In a small saucepan, heat coconut milk until warm.
2. Stir in gelatin and whisk until dissolved.
3. Add honey and vanilla extract, mixing well.
4. Pour into molds and refrigerate for at least 2 hours or until set.

**Tips:**

- Top with fresh berries or a sprinkle of unsweetened coconut flakes.
- Use agar-agar as a vegetarian substitute for gelatin.

**Nutritional Values:**
Calories: 130, Fat: 7g, Carbs: 18g, Protein: 2g, Sugar: 14g

**Nutritional Values:**
Calories: 90, Fat: 1g, Carbs: 18g, Protein: 6g, Sugar: 14g

# CHAPTER 11: MEAL PLANS

Starting a new diet can feel overwhelming, but having a solid meal plan can set you up for success.

The **7-DAY KICK-START & DETOX PLAN** serves as the perfect launch point for your journey with the Dr. Now 1200-Calorie Diet Plan. Designed to provide both nutritious and flavorful meals, this plan focuses on keeping calories low while delivering a satisfying eating experience.

In addition to balanced meals, we've placed special attention on hydration and detoxification by incorporating detox beverages that help cleanse and refresh your body. You'll find these detox drinks, rich in ingredients like lemon, ginger, mint, and turmeric, in a dedicated chapter (Chapter 9.1 Detox Elixirs) to support your daily hydration and help remove toxins naturally.

This plan not only kick-starts your diet but also helps your body reset and re-energize!

The **COMPLETE 30 – DAY MEAL PLAN** focuses on three main meals (breakfast, lunch, and dinner) that are nutritious, balanced, and rich in lean proteins, vegetables, and low-calorie complex carbohydrates.
Protein is emphasized to help maintain muscle mass, boost metabolism, and promote satiety throughout the day. It's also important to limit added sugars and refined carbs, which can spike blood sugar levels and increase hunger.

While **snacks or desserts are not included daily** to maintain a 1200-calorie limit, you can find **ideas for low-calorie options** in the chapters dedicated to snacks and desserts (Chapter 8 and Chapter 10).
Remember, this diet is about adopting a healthy lifestyle, not about punishment, so allowing yourself a small treat occasionally is perfectly fine.

Keep in mind that this plan should be tailored to your specific needs, and consulting with your healthcare provider is always recommended before starting any new diet.

Finally, remember that **any change can be challenging at first.** Stay motivated, celebrate your progress, and see each healthy choice as an investment in your long-term well-being.

# 11.1 THE 7-DAY KICKSTART & DETOX MEAL PLAN

## The 7-Day Kickstart Meal Plan
### DAY 1: FRESH START

**BREAKFAST:** Spinach and Mushroom Omelette - 200 kcal
Add 1 slice of whole wheat bread with 1 teaspoon almond butter - 100 kcal

**BEVERAGE:** Green Tea with Lemon

**LUNCH:** Grilled Chicken Salad - 250 kcal
Add 1 tablespoon sliced almonds -

40 kcal
Add 1 slice of whole wheat bread - 70 kcal

**DINNER:** Lentil and Vegetable Soup - 220 kcal
Add 1 cup cooked quinoa - 220 kcal

**BEVERAGE:** Lemon Mint Detox Water

**Total Calories Approx.:** 1100 kcal

## The 7-Day Kickstart Meal Plan
### DAY 2: KEEP IT GOING

**BREAKFAST:** Greek Yogurt Parfait - 240 kcal
Add 1 tablespoon chia seeds - 60 kcal
Add 1 small banana - 90 kcal

**BEVERAGE:** Lemon Ginger Water

**LUNCH:** Turkey Lettuce Wraps - 180 kcal

Add 1/2 avocado - 100 kcal
Add 1 small apple - 80 kcal

**DINNER:** Zucchini Noodles with Turkey Meatballs - 300 kcal
Add a small mixed salad with 1 tablespoon olive oil - 120 kcal

**BEVERAGE:** Cucumber Lime Detox Water

**Total Calories Approx.:** 1170 kcal

## The 7-Day Kickstart Meal Plan
### DAY 3: NOURISH AND ENERGIZE

**BREAKFAST:** Quinoa Breakfast Bowl - 280 kcal
Add 1 hard-boiled egg - 70 kcal

**BEVERAGE:** Green Tea with Lemon

**LUNCH:** Quinoa and Black Bean Bowl - 320 kcal
Add 1 slice of whole wheat bread - 70 kcal

**DINNER:** Baked Salmon with Asparagus - 300 kcal
Add 1 tablespoon olive oil for seasoning the asparagus - 120 kcal
Add 1 small baked sweet potato - 100 kcal

**BEVERAGE:** Lemon Mint Detox Water

**Total Calories Approx.:** 1160 kcal

## The 7-Day Kickstart Meal Plan
### DAY 4: MIDWEEK MOTIVATION

**BREAKFAST:** Avocado Toast - 180 kcal
Add 1 hard-boiled egg - 70 kcal
Add 1 small orange - 60 kcal

**BEVERAGE:** Lemon Ginger Water

**LUNCH:** Shrimp and Avocado Salad - 250 kcal
Add 1 slice of whole wheat bread with 1 teaspoon hummus - 80 kcal

**DINNER:** Broccoli and Tofu Stir-Fry - 200 kcal
Add 1 cup cooked brown rice - 200 kcal
Add a small mixed salad with 1 tablespoon olive oil - 120 kcal

**BEVERAGE:** Turmeric Ginger Tea

**Total Calories Approx.:** 1160 kcal

## The 7-Day Kickstart Meal Plan
### DAY 5: FUEL WITH FLAVOR

**BREAKFAST:** Berry Smoothie - 130 kcal
Add 1 tablespoon almond butter - 90 kcal
Add 1 slice of whole wheat bread - 70 kcal

**BEVERAGE:** Cucumber Lime Detox Water

**LUNCH:** Spinach and Feta Stuffed Chicken Breast - 300 kcal

Add 1 small baked sweet potato - 100 kcal
**DINNER:** Eggplant and Tomato Stew - 180 kcal
Add 1/2 cup cooked whole wheat couscous - 110 kcal
Add 1/2 avocado - 100 kcal

**BEVERAGE:** Green Tea with Lemon

**Total Calories Approx.:** 1080 kcal

## The 7-Day Kickstart Meal Plan
### DAY 6: KEEP PUSHING

**BREAKFAST:** Vegetable Frittata - 180 kcal
Add 1 slice of whole wheat toast - 70 kcal
Add 1 cup mixed berries - 60 kcal

**BEVERAGE:** Turmeric Ginger Tea

**LUNCH:** Mediterranean Chickpea Salad - 320 kcal
Add 1 tablespoon sunflower seeds - 50 kcal

Add 1 slice of whole wheat bread – 70 kcal

**DINNER:** Turkey and Spinach Stuffed Peppers - 250 kcal
Add 1 cup cooked brown rice - 200 kcal

**BEVERAGE:** Lemon Mint Detox Water

**Total Calories Approx.:** 1200 kcal

- **BREAKFAST:** Chia Pudding - 130 kcal
Add 1 tablespoon honey - 60 kcal
Add 1 small orange - 60 kcal

  **BEVERAGE:** Green Tea with Lemon

- **LUNCH:** Grilled Vegetable Wrap - 300 kcal
Add 1 tablespoon extra hummus - 40 kcal

Add 1 small apple - 80 kcal

- **DINNER:** Tofu and Vegetable Stir-Fry - 200 kcal
Add 1 cup cooked brown rice - 200 kcal
Add a small mixed salad with 1 tablespoon olive oil - 120 kcal

  **BEVERAGE:** Lemon Ginger Water

  **Total Calories Approx.:** 1190 kcal

## 11.2 THE COMPLETE 30-DAY MEAL PLAN:

| 30-Day Meal Plan |
| --- |
| **DAY 1:** |

**BREAKFAST:** Greek Yogurt Parfait - 240 kcal
Add 1 slice whole wheat bread - 70 kcal

**LUNCH:** Grilled Chicken Salad - 250 kcal
Add 1 tablespoon sliced almonds - 40 kcal

**DINNER:** Zucchini Noodles with Turkey Meatballs - 300 kcal
Add a small mixed salad with 1 tablespoon olive oil - 120 kcal

**BEVERAGE:** Green Tea - 0 kcal

**Total Calories Approx.: 1020 kcal**

| 30-Day Meal Plan |
| --- |
| **DAY 2:** |

**BREAKFAST:** Scrambled Egg Whites with Veggies - 100 kcal
Add 1 slice whole wheat bread - 70 kcal
**LUNCH:** Turkey Lettuce Wraps - 180 kcal
Add 1/2 avocado - 100 kcal
**DINNER:** Baked Salmon with Asparagus - 300 kcal

Add 1 small baked sweet potato - 130 kcal

**BEVERAGE:** Lemon Water - 0 kcal

**Total Calories Approx.:** 1010 kcal

## 30-Day Meal Plan
### DAY 3:

**BREAKFAST:** Berry Smoothie - 130 kcal
Add 1 tablespoon almond butter - 90 kcal
**LUNCH:** Quinoa and Black Bean Bowl - 320 kcal
Add 1 slice whole wheat bread - 70 kcal

**DINNER:** Shrimp Stir-Fry with Broccoli - 250 kcal
Add 1/2 cup cooked brown rice - 110 kcal

**BEVERAGE:** Herbal Tea - 0 kcal

**Total Calories Approx.: 1050 kcal**

## 30-Day Meal Plan
### DAY 4:

**BREAKFAST:** Avocado Toast - 180 kcal
Add 1 hard-boiled egg - 70 kcal
**LUNCH:** Grilled Chicken and Vegetable Skewers - 250 kcal
Add 1 slice whole wheat bread - 70 kcal
**DINNER:** Eggplant and Tomato Stew - 180 kcal

Add 1/2 cup couscous - 110 kcal
Add 1 tablespoon olive oil to the stew - 120 kcal

**BEVERAGE:** Unsweetened Iced Tea - 0 kcal

**Total Calories Approx.: 1080 kcal**

## 30-Day Meal Plan
### DAY 5:

**BREAKFAST:** Almond Butter Banana Toast - 220 kcal
Add 1 small orange - 60 kcal
**LUNCH:** Lemon Garlic Shrimp Pasta - 300 kcal
Add a small mixed salad with 1 tablespoon olive oil - 120 kcal

**DINNER:** Cauliflower Rice Stir-Fry - 200 kcal
Add 1/2 cup cooked brown rice - 110 kcal

**BEVERAGE:** Sparkling Water - 0 kcal

**Total Calories Approx.: 1010 kcal**

## 30-Day Meal Plan
### DAY 6:

**BREAKFAST:** Vegetable Frittata - 180 kcal
Add 1 slice whole wheat toast - 70 kcal
**LUNCH:** Mediterranean Chickpea Salad - 320 kcal
Add 1 tablespoon sunflower seeds - 50 kcal

**DINNER:** Turkey Chili - 300 kcal
Add a small mixed salad with 1 tablespoon olive oil - 120 kcal

**BEVERAGE:** Black Coffee - 0 kcal

**Total Calories Approx.: 1040 kcal**

| 30-Day Meal Plan |
|:---:|
| **DAY 7:** |

| | |
|---|---|
| **BREAKFAST:** Quinoa Breakfast Bowl - 280 kcal<br>Add 1 hard-boiled egg - 70 kcal<br>**LUNCH:** Shrimp and Avocado Salad - 250 kcal<br>Add 1 slice whole wheat bread - 70 kcal<br>**DINNER:** Grilled Lemon Herb Chicken - 300 kcal | Add 1/2 cup cooked brown rice - 110 kcal<br><br>**BEVERAGE:** Herbal Tea - 0 kcal<br><br>**Total Calories Approx.:** 1080 kcal |

| 30-Day Meal Plan |
|:---:|
| **DAY 8:** |

| | |
|---|---|
| **BREAKFAST:** Spinach and Mushroom Omelette - 200 kcal<br>Add 1 slice whole wheat toast - 70 kcal<br>**LUNCH:** Turkey and Spinach Stuffed Peppers - 250 kcal<br>Add 1/2 cup cooked brown rice - 120 kcal<br>**DINNER:** Baked Cod with Lemon and Herbs - 160 kcal | Add a small mixed salad with 1 tablespoon olive oil - 120 kcal<br>Add 1 slice whole wheat bread - 70 kcal<br><br>**BEVERAGE:** Herbal Tea - 0 kcal<br><br>**Total Calories Approx.:** 990 kcal |

| 30-Day Meal Plan |
|:---:|
| **DAY 9:** |

| | |
|---|---|
| **BREAKFAST:** Cottage Cheese and Berry Bowl - 160 kcal<br>Add 1 slice whole wheat toast - 70 kcal<br>**LUNCH:** Grilled Vegetable Wrap - 300 kcal<br>Add 1 tablespoon hummus - 40 kcal<br>**DINNER:** Zucchini Noodles with Marinara Sauce - 120 kcal | Add 1 tablespoon Parmesan cheese - 20 kcal<br>Add 1/2 cup cooked brown rice - 110 kcal<br><br>**BEVERAGE:** Green Tea - 0 kcal<br><br>**Total Calories Approx.:** 1020 kcal |

| 30-Day Meal Plan |
|:---:|
| **DAY 10:** |

| | |
|---|---|
| **BREAKFAST:** Berry Smoothie - 130 kcal<br>Add 1 tablespoon almond butter - 90 kcal<br>**LUNCH:** Tofu and Vegetable Stir-Fry - 200 kcal<br>Add 1 slice whole wheat bread - 70 kcal<br>**DINNER:** Baked Salmon with Asparagus - 300 kcal | Add 1 small baked sweet potato - 130 kcal<br>Add a small mixed salad with 1 tablespoon olive oil - 120 kcal<br>**BEVERAGE:** Unsweetened Iced Tea - 0 kcal<br><br>**Total Calories Approx.:** 1040 kcal |

## 30-Day Meal Plan
### DAY 11:

**BREAKFAST:** Vegetable Frittata - 180 kcal
Add 1 slice whole wheat toast - 70 kcal
**LUNCH:** Quinoa and Black Bean Bowl - 320 kcal
Add 1 slice whole wheat bread - 70 kcal

**DINNER:** Grilled Lemon Herb Chicken - 300 kcal
Add a small mixed salad with 1 tablespoon olive oil - 120 kcal

**BEVERAGE:** Lemon Water - 0 kcal

**Total Calories Approx.:** 1060 kcal

## 30-Day Meal Plan
### DAY 12:

**BREAKFAST:** Almond Butter Banana Toast - 220 kcal
Add 1 small orange - 60 kcal
**LUNCH:** Turkey Lettuce Wraps - 180 kcal
Add 1/2 avocado - 100 kcal
**DINNER:** Shrimp Stir-Fry with Broccoli - 250 kcal

Add 1/2 cup cooked brown rice – 110 kcal
Add a small mixed salad with 1 tablespoon olive oil - 120 kcal

**BEVERAGE:** Herbal Tea - 0 kcal

**Total Calories Approx.:** 1040 kcal

## 30-Day Meal Plan
### DAY 13:

**BREAKFAST:** Quinoa Breakfast Bowl - 280 kcal
Add 1 hard-boiled egg - 70 kcal
**LUNCH:** Lemon Garlic Shrimp Pasta - 300 kcal
Add a small mixed salad with 1 tablespoon olive oil - 120 kcal
**DINNER:** Grilled Chicken and Vegetable Skewers - 250 kcal

Add 1/2 cup cooked brown rice - 110 kcal

**BEVERAGE:** Green Tea - 0 kcal

**Total Calories Approx.:** 1130 kcal

## 30-Day Meal Plan
### DAY 14:

**BREAKFAST:** Chia Pudding with Almond Milk - 140 kcal
Add 1 tablespoon honey - 60 kcal
**LUNCH:** Quinoa and Black Bean Bowl - 320 kcal
Add 1 slice whole wheat bread - 70 kcal

**DINNER:** Turkey Chili - 300 kcal
Add a small mixed salad with 1 tablespoon olive oil - 120 kcal
**BEVERAGE:** Sparkling Water - 0 kcal

**Total Calories Approx.:** 1010 kcal

## 30-Day Meal Plan
### DAY 15:

**BREAKFAST:** Scrambled Egg Whites with Veggies - 100 kcal
Add 1 slice whole wheat bread - 70 kcal
**LUNCH:** Spinach and Feta Stuffed Chicken Breast - 300 kcal
Add 1/2 cup cooked brown rice - 120 kcal
**DINNER:** Baked Tilapia with Roasted Vegetables - 160 kcal

Add 1 slice whole wheat bread - 70 kcal
Add a small mixed salad with 1 tablespoon olive oil - 120 kcal

**BEVERAGE:** Lemon Water - 0 kcal

**Total Calories Approx.:** 1040 kcal

## 30-Day Meal Plan
### DAY 16:

**BREAKFAST:** Vegetable Frittata - 180 kcal
Add 1 slice whole wheat toast - 70 kcal
**LUNCH:** Mediterranean Chickpea Salad - 320 kcal
Add 1 tablespoon sunflower seeds - 50 kcal
**DINNER:** Baked Cod with Lemon and Herbs - 160 kcal

Add 1/2 cup cooked brown rice - 110 kcal
Add a small mixed salad with 1 tablespoon olive oil - 120 kcal

**BEVERAGE:** Green Tea - 0 kcal

**Total Calories Approx.:** 1010 kcal

## 30-Day Meal Plan
### DAY 17:

**BREAKFAST:** Greek Yogurt Parfait - 240 kcal
Add 1 slice whole wheat bread - 70 kcal
**LUNCH:** Turkey and Spinach Stuffed Peppers - 250 kcal
Add 1/2 cup cooked brown rice - 120 kcal
**DINNER:** Zucchini Noodles with Turkey Meatballs - 300 kcal

Add a small mixed salad with 1 tablespoon olive oil - 120 kcal

**BEVERAGE:** Herbal Tea - 0 kcal

**Total Calories Approx.:** 1100 kcal

## 30-Day Meal Plan
### DAY 18:

**BREAKFAST:** Avocado Toast - 180 kcal
Add 1 hard-boiled egg - 70 kcal
**LUNCH:** Grilled Vegetable Wrap - 300 kcal
Add 1 tablespoon hummus - 40 kcal
**DINNER:** Lentil and Vegetable Soup - 220 kcal

Add 1 slice whole wheat bread - 70 kcal
Add 1 tablespoon olive oil - 120 kcal

**BEVERAGE:** Lemon Water - 0 kcal

**Total Calories Approx.:** 1000 kcal

## 30-Day Meal Plan
### DAY 19:

**BREAKFAST:** Quinoa Breakfast Bowl - 280 kcal
Add 1 hard-boiled egg - 70 kcal
**LUNCH:** Grilled Chicken Salad - 250 kcal
Add 1 tablespoon sliced almonds - 40 kcal
**DINNER:** Salmon with Asparagus - 300 kcal

Add a small baked sweet potato - 130 kcal

**BEVERAGE:** Unsweetened Iced Tea - 0 kcal

**Total Calories Approx.:** 1070 kcal

## 30-Day Meal Plan
### DAY 20:

**BREAKFAST:** Almond Butter Banana Toast - 220 kcal
Add 1 small orange - 60 kcal
**LUNCH:** Grilled Chicken and Vegetable Skewers - 250 kcal
Add 1 slice whole wheat bread - 70 kcal
**DINNER:** Shrimp Stir-Fry with Broccoli - 250 kcal

Add 1/2 cup cooked brown rice - 110 kcal
Add a small mixed salad with 1 tablespoon olive oil - 120 kcal

**BEVERAGE:** Green Tea - 0 kcal

**Total Calories Approx.:** 1080 kcal

## 30-Day Meal Plan
### DAY 21:

**BREAKFAST:** Chia Pudding with Almond Milk - 140 kcal
Add 1 tablespoon honey - 60 kcal
**LUNCH:** Tuna and White Bean Salad - 250 kcal
Add 1 slice whole wheat bread - 70 kcal
**DINNER:** Baked Chicken with Cauliflower Mash - 300 kcal

Add a small mixed salad with 1 tablespoon olive oil - 120 kcal

**BEVERAGE:** Sparkling Water - 0 kcal

**Total Calories Approx.:** 1040 kcal

## 30-Day Meal Plan
### DAY 22:

**BREAKFAST:** Spinach and Mushroom Omelette - 200 kcal
Add 1 slice whole wheat toast - 70 kcal
**LUNCH:** Quinoa and Black Bean Bowl - 320 kcal
Add 1 slice whole wheat bread - 70 kcal

**DINNER:** Turkey and Spinach Meatballs - 300 kcal
Add 1/2 cup cooked brown rice - 120 kcal

**BEVERAGE:** Herbal Tea - 0 kcal

**Total Calories Approx.:** 1080 kcal

## 30-Day Meal Plan
### DAY 23:

**BREAKFAST:** Greek Yogurt Parfait - 240 kcal
Add 1 slice whole wheat bread - 70 kcal
**LUNCH:** Shrimp and Avocado Salad - 250 kcal
Add 1/2 avocado - 100 kcal
**DINNER:** Grilled Lemon Herb Chicken - 300 kcal

Add a small mixed salad with 1 tablespoon olive oil - 120 kcal

**BEVERAGE:** Lemon Water - 0 kcal

**Total Calories Approx.:** 1080 kcal

## 30-Day Meal Plan
### DAY 24:

**BREAKFAST:** Scrambled Egg Whites with Veggies - 100 kcal
Add 1 slice whole wheat bread - 70 kcal
**LUNCH:** Grilled Vegetable Wrap - 300 kcal
Add 1 tablespoon hummus - 40 kcal
**DINNER:** Baked Tilapia with Roasted Vegetables - 160 kcal

Add 1 slice whole wheat bread - 70 kcal
Add a small mixed salad with 1 tablespoon olive oil - 120 kcal

**BEVERAGE:** Green Tea - 0 kcal

**Total Calories Approx.:** 1010 kcal

## 30-Day Meal Plan
### DAY 25:

**BREAKFAST:** Vegetable Frittata - 180 kcal
Add 1 slice whole wheat toast - 70 kcal
**LUNCH:** Mediterranean Chickpea Salad - 320 kcal
Add 1 tablespoon sunflower seeds - 50 kcal
**DINNER:** Eggplant and Tomato Stew - 180 kcal

Add 1/2 cup cooked couscous - 120 kcal
Add a small mixed salad with 1 tablespoon olive oil - 120 kcal

**BEVERAGE:** Sparkling Water - 0 kcal

**Total Calories Approx.:** 1040 kcal

## 30-Day Meal Plan
### DAY 26:

**BREAKFAST:** Avocado Toast - 180 kcal
Add 1 hard-boiled egg - 70 kcal
**LUNCH:** Quinoa and Black Bean Bowl - 320 kcal
Add 1 slice whole wheat bread - 70 kcal
**DINNER:** Baked Cod with Lemon and Herbs - 160 kcal

Add 1/2 cup cooked brown rice - 110 kcal
Add a small mixed salad with 1 tablespoon olive oil - 120 kcal

**BEVERAGE:** Herbal Tea - 0 kcal

**Total Calories Approx.:** 1030 kcal

| 30-Day Meal Plan |
|---|
| **DAY 27:** |

**BREAKFAST:** Almond Butter Banana Toast - 220 kcal
Add 1 small orange - 60 kcal
**LUNCH:** Grilled Chicken Salad - 250 kcal
Add 1 tablespoon sliced almonds - 40 kcal
**DINNER:** Turkey and Spinach Meatballs - 300 kcal

Add 1/2 cup cooked brown rice - 120 kcal
Add a small mixed salad with 1 tablespoon olive oil - 120 kcal

**BEVERAGE:** Green Tea - 0 kcal

**Total Calories Approx.:** 1130 kcal

| 30-Day Meal Plan |
|---|
| **DAY 28:** |

**BREAKFAST:** Greek Yogurt Parfait - 240 kcal
Add 1 slice whole wheat bread - 70 kcal
**LUNCH:** Tuna and White Bean Salad - 250 kcal
Add 1 slice whole wheat bread - 70 kcal

**DINNER:** Baked Chicken with Cauliflower Mash - 300 kcal
Add a small mixed salad with 1 tablespoon olive oil - 120 kcal

**BEVERAGE:** Lemon Water - 0 kcal

**Total Calories Approx.:** 1050 kcal

| 30-Day Meal Plan |
|---|
| **DAY 29:** |

**BREAKFAST:** Quinoa Breakfast Bowl - 280 kcal
Add 1 hard-boiled egg - 70 kcal
**LUNCH:** Shrimp and Avocado Salad - 250 kcal
Add 1 slice whole wheat bread - 70 kcal
**DINNER:** Grilled Chicken and Vegetable Skewers - 250 kcal

Add 1/2 cup cooked brown rice - 120 kcal

**BEVERAGE:** Unsweetened Iced Tea - 0 kcal

**Total Calories Approx.:** 1040 kcal

| 30-Day Meal Plan |
|---|
| **DAY 30:** |

**BREAKFAST:** Vegetable Frittata - 180 kcal
Add 1 slice whole wheat toast - 70 kcal
**LUNCH:** Mediterranean Chickpea Salad - 320 kcal
Add 1 tablespoon sunflower seeds - 50 kcal

**DINNER:** Salmon with Asparagus - 300 kcal
Add 1 small baked sweet potato - 130 kcal

**BEVERAGE:** Herbal Tea - 0 kcal

**Total Calories Approx.:** 1050 kcal

# KITCHEN
## CONVERSION CHART

| CUP | TBSP | TSP | OZ | ML |
|---|---|---|---|---|
| 1 C | 16 TBSP | 48 TSP | 8 OZ | 240 ML |
| 3/4 C | 12 TBSP | 36 TSP | 6 OZ | 180 ML |
| 2/3 C | 10 TBSP + 2 TSP 1/2 | 32 TSP | $5^{1/3}$ OZ | 160 ML |
| 1/2 C | 8 TBSP | 24 TSP | 4 OZ | 120 ML |
| 1/3 C | 5 TBSP + 1TSP 1/8 | 16 TSP | $2^{2/3}$ OZ | 80 ML |
| 1/4 C | 4 TBSP | 12 TSP | 2 OZ | 60 ML |
| 1/6 C | 2 TBSP + 2 TSP | 8 TSP | $1^{1/3}$ OZ | 40 ML |
| 1/8 C | 2 TBSP | 6 TSP | 1 OZ | 30 ML |
| 1/16 C | 1 TBSP | 3 TSP | 1/2 OZ | 15 ML |

BUTTER
1 STICK
=1/2 CUP

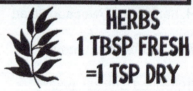
HERBS
1 TBSP FRESH
=1 TSP DRY

# CONCLUSION

As we reach the end of this book, it's time to take a moment and acknowledge the incredible journey you've embarked on. You've done more than just read through recipes and strategies; you've taken powerful steps toward transforming your life, following the principles laid out by Dr. Nowzaradan.

You have learned how to nourish your body with wholesome, balanced meals, and how to navigate the challenges of cravings and setbacks. Each recipe you have tried, each strategy you've implemented, has been like planting a seed in your personal garden of wellness. And now, you are beginning to see the fruits of your labor—whether it's weight loss, increased energy, or a renewed sense of confidence and control over your health.

As you continue to embrace Dr. Now's approach, do not be afraid to make it your own. Adapt the recipes to suit your tastes, experiment with new ingredients, and keep exploring flavors that excite you. The goal is to create a sustainable, enjoyable way of eating that you can stick to for the long haul.

We hope that this book has served as a toolkit, a roadmap, and a source of inspiration to help you achieve your health goals. The lessons and skills you have gained here are just the beginning. Keep pushing forward, keep experimenting in the kitchen, and most importantly, keep believing in yourself. You have the power to create the life you want—one meal, one workout, one day at a time.

The future is yours to shape, and with the knowledge and tools you have gathered here, you're more than equipped to make it a healthy and fulfilling one.

XOXO *Magda Tangy*

# A GIFT FOR YOU: *The Weight Loss Success Kit*

Thank you for choosing
**"Dr. Now 1200 Calorie Diet Plan"**

As a token of our appreciation, we invite you to download your free bonus.

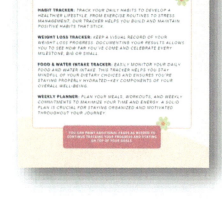

**"WEIGHT LOSS SUCCESS KIT"**

**Scan the QR code below to get your free gift:**

## We Value Your Feedback!

Your experience matters to us, and we would love to hear your thoughts. If you enjoyed the book or found it helpful, please consider leaving a review on Amazon.com. Your feedback not only helps us improve but also assists other readers in making informed choices.

Thank you for your support!

*Magda Tangy*